SUMMARY

THE LEARNING HEALTH SYSTEM SERIES

ROUNDTABLE ON VALUE & SCIENCE-DRIVEN HEALTH CARE

THE HEALTHCARE IMPERATIVE
Lowering Costs and Improving Outcomes

Workshop Series Summary

Pierre L. Yong, Robert S. Saunders, and LeighAnne Olsen, *Editors*

INSTITUTE OF MEDICINE
OF THE NATIONAL ACADEMIES

THE NATIONAL ACADEMIES PRESS
Washington, D.C.
www.nap.edu

THE NATIONAL ACADEMIES PRESS   500 Fifth Street, N.W.   Washington, DC 20001

NOTICE: The project that is the subject of this report was approved by the Governing Board of the National Research Council, whose members are drawn from the councils of the National Academy of Sciences, the National Academy of Engineering, and the Institute of Medicine.

This project was supported by the Peter G. Peterson Foundation. Any opinions, findings, conclusions, or recommendations expressed in this publication are those of the author(s) and do not necessarily reflect the view of the organizations or agencies that provided support for this project.

International Standard Book Number-13: 978-0-309-14433-9
International Standard Book Number-10: 0-309-14433-7

Additional copies of this Summary are available in limited quantities from the Institute of Medicine, 500 Fifth Street, N.W., Washington, DC 20001.

Copies of *The Healthcare Imperative,* from which this Summary has been extracted, are available from the National Academies Press, 500 Fifth Street, N.W., Lockbox 285, Washington, DC 20055; (800) 624-6242 or (202) 334-3313 (in the Washington metropolitan area); Internet, http://www.nap.edu.

For more information about the Institute of Medicine, visit the IOM home page at: **www.iom.edu.**

The serpent has been a symbol of long life, healing, and knowledge among almost all cultures and religions since the beginning of recorded history. The serpent adopted as a logotype by the Institute of Medicine is a relief carving from ancient Greece, now held by the Staatliche Museen in Berlin.

Suggested citation: IOM (Institute of Medicine). 2010. *The Healthcare Imperative: Lowering Costs and Improving Outcomes: Workshop Series Summary.* Washington, DC: The National Academies Press.

"Knowing is not enough; we must apply. Willing is not enough; we must do."
—Goethe

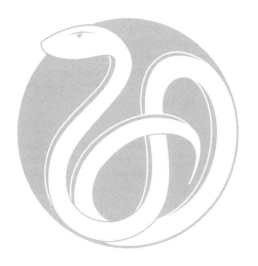

INSTITUTE OF MEDICINE
OF THE NATIONAL ACADEMIES

Advising the Nation. Improving Health.

THE NATIONAL ACADEMIES
Advisers to the Nation on Science, Engineering, and Medicine

The **National Academy of Sciences** is a private, nonprofit, self-perpetuating society of distinguished scholars engaged in scientific and engineering research, dedicated to the furtherance of science and technology and to their use for the general welfare. Upon the authority of the charter granted to it by the Congress in 1863, the Academy has a mandate that requires it to advise the federal government on scientific and technical matters. Dr. Ralph J. Cicerone is president of the National Academy of Sciences.

The **National Academy of Engineering** was established in 1964, under the charter of the National Academy of Sciences, as a parallel organization of outstanding engineers. It is autonomous in its administration and in the selection of its members, sharing with the National Academy of Sciences the responsibility for advising the federal government. The National Academy of Engineering also sponsors engineering programs aimed at meeting national needs, encourages education and research, and recognizes the superior achievements of engineers. Dr. Charles M. Vest is president of the National Academy of Engineering.

The **Institute of Medicine** was established in 1970 by the National Academy of Sciences to secure the services of eminent members of appropriate professions in the examination of policy matters pertaining to the health of the public. The Institute acts under the responsibility given to the National Academy of Sciences by its congressional charter to be an adviser to the federal government and, upon its own initiative, to identify issues of medical care, research, and education. Dr. Harvey V. Fineberg is president of the Institute of Medicine.

The **National Research Council** was organized by the National Academy of Sciences in 1916 to associate the broad community of science and technology with the Academy's purposes of furthering knowledge and advising the federal government. Functioning in accordance with general policies determined by the Academy, the Council has become the principal operating agency of both the National Academy of Sciences and the National Academy of Engineering in providing services to the government, the public, and the scientific and engineering communities. The Council is administered jointly by both Academies and the Institute of Medicine. Dr. Ralph J. Cicerone and Dr. Charles M. Vest are chair and vice chair, respectively, of the National Research Council.

www.national-academies.org

ROUNDTABLE ON VALUE & SCIENCE-DRIVEN HEALTH CARE[1]

Denis A. Cortese (*Chair*), Emeritus President and Chief Executive Officer, Mayo Clinic; Foundation Professor, ASU

Donald Berwick, Administrator, Centers for Medicare & Medicaid Services (*ex officio*)

David Blumenthal, National Coordinator, Office of the National Coordinator for Health IT (*ex officio*)

Bruce G. Bodaken, Chairman, President, and Chief Executive Officer, Blue Shield of California

David R. Brennan, Chief Executive Officer, AstraZeneca PLC

Paul Chew, Chief Science Officer and CMO, sanofi-aventis U.S., Inc.

Carolyn M. Clancy, Director, Agency for Healthcare Research and Quality (*ex officio*)

Michael J. Critelli, Former Executive Chairman, Pitney Bowes, Inc.

Helen Darling, President, National Business Group on Health

Thomas R. Frieden, Director, Centers for Disease Control and Prevention (*designee*: **Chesley Richards**) (*ex officio*)

Gary L. Gottlieb, President and CEO, Partners HealthCare System

James A. Guest, President, Consumers Union

George C. Halvorson, Chairman and Chief Executive Officer, Kaiser Permanente

Margaret A. Hamburg, Commissioner, Food and Drug Administration (*ex officio*)

Carmen Hooker Odom, President, Milbank Memorial Fund

Ardis Hoven, Professor of Medicine, University of Kentucky; Chair-elect, American Medical Association

Brent James, Chief Quality Officer and Executive Director, Institute for Health Care Delivery Research, Intermountain Healthcare

Michael M. E. Johns, Chancellor, Emory University

Craig Jones, Director, Vermont Blueprint for Health

Cato T. Laurencin, Vice President for Health Affairs, Dean of the School of Medicine, University of Connecticut

Stephen P. MacMillan, President and Chief Executive Officer, Stryker

Mark B. McClellan, Director, Engelberg Center for Healthcare Reform, The Brookings Institution

Sheri S. McCoy, Worldwide Chairman, Johnson & Johnson Pharmaceuticals Group

Elizabeth G. Nabel, President, Brigham and Women's Hospital

---

[1] Formerly the Roundtable on Evidence-Based Medicine. IOM forums and roundtables do not issue, review, or approve individual documents. The responsibility for the published workshop summary rests with the workshop rapporteurs and the institution.

Mary D. Naylor, Professor and Director of Center for Transitions in Health, University of Pennsylvania

Peter Neupert, Corporate Vice President, Health Solutions Group, Microsoft Corporation

Nancy H. Nielsen, Past President, American Medical Association

William D. Novelli, Former CEO, AARP; Professor, Georgetown University

Jonathan B. Perlin, Chief Medical Officer and President, Clinical Services, HCA, Inc.

Robert A. Petzel, Under Secretary, Veterans Health Administration (*ex officio*)

Richard Platt, Professor and Chair, Harvard Medical School and Harvard Pilgrim Health Care

John C. Rother, Group Executive Officer, AARP

John W. Rowe, Professor, Mailman School of Public Health, Columbia University

Susan Shurin, Acting Director, National Heart, Lung, and Blood Institute (*ex officio*)

Mark D. Smith, President and CEO, California HealthCare Foundation

George P. Taylor, Assistant Secretary for Health Affairs (Acting), Department of Defense (*designee*: Michael Dinneen) (*ex officio*)

Reed D. Tuckson, Executive VP and Chief of Medical Affairs, UnitedHealth Group

Frances M. Visco, President, National Breast Cancer Coalition

Workshop Planning Committee

Arnold Milstein (*Chair*), Pacific Business Group on Health
Kathleen Buto, Johnson & Johnson
Robert S. Galvin, Global Healthcare/General Electric
Paul B. Ginsburg, Center for Studying Health System Change
Eric Jensen, McKinsey Global Institute
James Mathews, Medicare Payment Advisory Commission
Nancy H. Nielsen, American Medical Association
Steven D. Pearson, Institute for Clinical and Economic Review
Gail Shearer, Consumers Union
Reed V. Tuckson, UnitedHealth Group

Roundtable Staff

Christie Bell, Financial Associate
Patrick Burke, Financial Associate (through December 2009)
Jane Fredell, Program Assistant (through September 2009)
China Dickerson, Program Assistant (through November 2009)

Chanda Ijames, Program Assistant (through December 2009)
J. Michael McGinnis, Senior Scholar and Executive Director
Claudia Grossmann, Program Officer
LeighAnne Olsen, Program Officer (through June 2010)
Brian Powers, Program Assistant
Robert Saunders, Program Officer
Pierre L. Yong, Program Officer (through May 2010)
Kate Vasconi, Senior Program Assistant
Catherine Zweig, Senior Program Assistant (through June 2010)

Reviewers

This report has been reviewed in draft form by individuals chosen for their diverse perspectives and technical expertise, in accordance with procedures approved by the National Research Council's Report Review Committee. The purpose of this independent review is to provide candid and critical comments that will assist the institution in making its published report as sound as possible and to ensure that the report meets institutional standards for objectivity, evidence, and responsiveness to the study charge. The review comments and draft manuscript remain confidential to protect the integrity of the process. We wish to thank the following individuals for their review of this report:

Helen Darling, National Business Group on Health
Robert S. Mecklenberg, Virginia Mason Medical Center
Sheila Smith, Office of the Actuary
Sean Tunis, Center for Medical Technology Policy

Although the reviewers listed above have provided many constructive comments and suggestions, they were not asked to endorse the final draft of the report before its release. The review of this report was overseen by **Floyd Bloom**. Appointed by the National Research Council and the Institute of Medicine, he was responsible for making certain that an independent examination of this report was carried out in accordance with institutional procedures and that all review comments were carefully considered. Responsibility for the final content of this report rests entirely with the editors and the institution.

Institute of Medicine
Roundtable on Value & Science-Driven Health Care[1]
Charter and Vision Statement

The Institute of Medicine's Roundtable on Value & Science-Driven Health Care has been convened to help transform the way evidence on clinical effectiveness is generated and used to improve health and health care. Participants have set a goal that, by the year 2020, 90 percent of clinical decisions will be supported by accurate, timely, and up-to-date clinical information, and will reflect the best available evidence. Roundtable members will work with their colleagues to identify the issues not being adequately addressed, the nature of the barriers and possible solutions, and the priorities for action, and will marshal the resources of the sectors represented on the Roundtable to work for sustained public-private cooperation for change.

* *

The Institute of Medicine's Roundtable on Value & Science-Driven Health Care has been convened to help transform the way evidence on clinical effectiveness is generated and used to improve health and health care. We seek the development of a *learning health system* that is designed to generate and apply the best evidence for the collaborative healthcare choices of each patient and provider; to drive the process of discovery as a natural outgrowth of patient care, and to ensure innovation, quality, safety, and value in health care.

Vision: Our vision is for a healthcare system that draws on the best evidence to provide the care most appropriate to each patient, emphasizes prevention and health promotion, delivers the most value, adds to learning throughout the delivery of care, and leads to improvements in the nation's health.

Goal: By the year 2020, 90 percent of clinical decisions will be supported by accurate, timely, and up-to-date clinical information, and will reflect the best available evidence. We feel that this presents a tangible focus for progress toward our vision, that Americans ought to expect at least this level of performance, that it should be feasible with existing resources and emerging tools, and that measures can be developed to track and stimulate progress.

Context: As unprecedented developments in the diagnosis, treatment, and long-term management of disease bring Americans closer than ever to the promise of personalized health care, we are faced with similarly unprecedented challenges to identify and deliver the care most appropriate for individual needs and conditions. Care that is important is often not delivered. Care that is delivered is often not important. In part, this is due to our failure to apply the evidence we have about the medical care that is most effective—a failure related to shortfalls in provider knowledge and accountability, inadequate care coordination and support, lack of insurance, poorly aligned payment incentives, and misplaced patient expectations. Increasingly, it is also a result of our

---

[1] Formerly the Roundtable on Evidence-Based Medicine.

limited capacity for timely generation of evidence on the relative effectiveness, efficiency, and safety of available and emerging interventions. Improving the value of the return on our healthcare investment is a vital imperative that will require much greater capacity to evaluate high priority clinical interventions, stronger links between clinical research and practice, and reorientation of the incentives to apply new insights. We must quicken our efforts to position evidence development and application as natural outgrowths of clinical care—to foster health care that learns.

Approach: The IOM Roundtable on Value & Science-Driven Health Care serves as a forum to facilitate the collaborative assessment and action around issues central to achieving the vision and goal stated. The challenges are myriad and include issues that must be addressed to improve evidence development, evidence application, and the capacity to advance progress on both dimensions. To address these challenges, as leaders in their fields, Roundtable members will work with their colleagues to identify the issues not being adequately addressed, the nature of the barriers and possible solutions, and the priorities for action, and will marshal the resources of the sectors represented on the Roundtable to work for sustained public-private cooperation for change.

Activities include collaborative exploration of new and expedited approaches to assessing the effectiveness of diagnostic and treatment interventions, better use of the patient care experience to generate evidence on effectiveness, identification of assessment priorities, and communication strategies to enhance provider and patient understanding and support for interventions proven to work best and deliver value in health care.

Core concepts and principles: For the purpose of the Roundtable activities, we define science-driven health care broadly to mean that, *to the greatest extent possible, the decisions that shape the health and health care of Americans—by patients, providers, payers, and policymakers alike—will be grounded on a reliable evidence base, will account appropriately for individual variation in patient needs, and will support the generation of new insights on clinical effectiveness.* Evidence is generally considered to be information from clinical experience that has met some established test of validity, and the appropriate standard is determined according to the requirements of the intervention and clinical circumstance. Processes that involve the development and use of evidence should be accessible and transparent to all stakeholders.

A common commitment to certain principles and priorities guides the activities of the Roundtable and its members, including the commitment to: the right health care for each person; putting the best evidence into practice; establishing the effectiveness, efficiency, and safety of medical care delivered; building constant measurement into our healthcare investments; the establishment of healthcare data as a public good; shared responsibility distributed equitably across stakeholders, both public and private; collaborative stakeholder involvement in priority setting; transparency in the execution of activities and reporting of results; and subjugation of individual political or stakeholder perspectives in favor of the common good.

Foreword

Health reform is driven by the needs of the 47 million uninsured in this country and is also propelled by the central issue of cost. Escalating national healthcare expenditures engulf a rapidly enlarging fraction of the federal budget. Businesses pass part of the soaring costs on to their employees in the form of rising health insurance premiums. Families struggle to pay their healthcare bills, and many have delayed seeking necessary and important care.

Since 2006, the Institute of Medicine has assembled the diverse leadership across the health care system—including patient and consumer, provider, manufacturer, payer, research and policy representatives—under the auspices of our Roundtable on Value & Science-Driven Health Care (formerly the Roundtable on Evidence-Based Medicine) to engage the pressing issues confronting the U.S. healthcare delivery system today. Under the guidance of its membership, the Roundtable developed the vision of a learning health system, one in which evidence development is not merely an occasional byproduct of health care, but one in which evidence capture and analysis, as well as its application, is systematically structured as an integral and natural component of the care process. Building on its efforts to enhance the value obtained from health expenditures and with the generous support of the Peter G. Peterson Foundation, the Roundtable convened stakeholders from across the healthcare field in a series of four 2-day meetings, titled The Healthcare Imperative: Lowering Costs and Improving Outcomes. These sessions were devoted to understanding the sources of excess costs in health care, reviewing what is known about ways to reduce the excess, and identifying policy solutions.

This summary highlights the presentations and discussions from these workshops, delving into the major causes of excess spending, waste, and inefficiency in health care; considering the strategies that might reduce per capita health spending in the United States while improving health outcomes and preserving innovation; and exploring the policy options that would facilitate those strategies. The ideas and observations throughout this volume are offered in the belief that health reform, now and in the future, will benefit from identifying actionable options to lower healthcare costs in ways that maximize value.

I would like to extend my personal thanks especially to the Peter G. Peterson Foundation and its President, David Walker, to the Planning Committee assembled for the series, to the Roundtable membership for their continued leadership and commitment to advancing health care in this nation, and to the Roundtable staff for their contributions in coordinating and supporting the meeting series and ongoing Roundtable activities.

Harvey V. Fineberg, M.D., Ph.D.
President, Institute of Medicine

Preface

Stimulated by the challenges facing our nation as healthcare expenditures continue to soar and threaten our fiscal future, the four-part workshop series The Healthcare Imperative: Lowering Costs and Improving Outcomes, supported by the Peter G. Peterson Foundation, explored in detail the sources and implications of waste and excess cost in health care, as well as the strategies and policies necessary to address the issues. This volume summarizes the workshops, which were convened in May, July, September, and December of 2009 by the Institute of Medicine (IOM) Roundtable on Value & Science-Driven Health Care (formerly the Roundtable on Evidence-Based Medicine), as part of its *Learning Health System* workshop series. These meetings offered a forum for the broad spectrum of stakeholders in health to discuss the range of issues pertinent to reducing health spending without compromising health status, quality of care, or valued innovation. The discussion summary and its related presentations reflect the contributions of experts from multiple sectors involved in leadership, policy, practice, and innovation on behalf of better value in health care.

Guided by its membership, the vision of the IOM Roundtable on Value & Science-Driven Health Care is to catalyze the development of a *learning health system*—a system in which the processes and systems utilized by the healthcare system enable both the natural delivery of best care practices and the real-time generation and application of new evidence. With the support of senior leadership from the country's key healthcare sectors, the Roundtable has furthered its vision through collaborative initiatives, including public workshops and published proceedings. This workshop series emerged from prior work of the Roundtable on value in health care, as well as the ongoing dialogue on healthcare reform, and provided a forum for stakeholders to discuss their perspectives and to identify ideas and areas for further consideration.

The contributions of the workshop discussions to better understanding have been conceptual, quantitative, and qualitative. Conceptually, the approach fashioned by the Planning Committee grouped the sources of excess costs in health care into six domains: unnecessary services (volume), services delivered inefficiently, prices that are too high, excessive administrative costs, missed prevention opportunities, and fraud. Except for the last, the sessions organized by the Committee for the first workshop reviewed these domains in detail, and, while much work remains, the workshop presentations have offered a substantially enhanced understanding of the nature and size of the problems in each of those domains. Two things are clear: (1) each is an important contributor to excessive healthcare costs, and (2) the amount of excessive costs incurred from each is tremendous.

In discussions about potential cost control strategies and policy options, key levers for change were identified and considered in the second and third workshops, as vehicles for initiatives of particular policy relevance, including payment transformation, governance streamlining, transparency, knowledge development, care system redesign, and community health capacity. The nature, barriers, and potential impact of the various measures were extensively explored. At the request of the Planning Committee, a fourth workshop was scheduled to focus solely on the Series' motivating proposition: reducing healthcare costs by 10 percent within 10 years, without compromising health outcomes or valued innovation.

Throughout the progression of the meetings, a number of opportunities and challenges were also identified around which the engagement of stakeholders such as those represented on the Roundtable, might be especially important and facilitative. These issues will be explored through future workshops, commissioned papers, collaborative activities, and public communication efforts.

We are especially indebted to the members of the Planning Committee, which crafted this unusually productive and path-breaking discussion series. The members of this stellar group were: Arnold Milstein (Pacific Business Group on Health, Committee Chair), Kathleen Buto (Johnson & Johnson), Robert S. Galvin (Global Healthcare/General Electric), Paul B. Ginsburg (Center for Studying Health System Change), Eric Jensen (McKinsey Global Institute), James Mathews (Medicare Payment Advisory Commission), Nancy H. Nielsen (American Medical Association), Steven D. Pearson (Institute for Clinical and Economic Review), Gail Shearer (Consumers Union), and Reed V. Tuckson (UnitedHealth Group).

Multiple other individuals and organizations donated their valuable time toward the development of this publication. We naturally also acknowledge and offer strong appreciation for the contributors to this volume, for the care and thought that went into their analyses and presentations, for the ideas and observations they shared at the workshops, and for their contributions to this summary publication. In this respect, we should underscore that this volume contains a collection of individually authored papers and intends to convey only the views and beliefs of those participating in the workshops, not the express opinions of the Roundtable on Value & Science-Driven Health Care, its members, its sponsors, or the Institute of Medicine.

A number of Roundtable staff played instrumental roles in coordinating the workshops and translating the workshop proceedings into this summary, including Pierre L. Yong (the staff officer with primary responsibility), Catherine Zweig, LeighAnne Olsen, Kate Vasconi, Jane Fredell, China Dickerson, Chanda Ijames, Patrick Burke, Christie Bell, and Ruth Strommen. Franklin A. Cruz also contributed substantially to publication development. We would also like to thank Vilija Teel, Jordan Wyndelts, Michele de la Menardiere, and Jackie Turner for helping to coordinate the various aspects of review, production, and publication.

Clearly, successfully addressing the challenges of lowering healthcare expenditures while preserving outcomes and innovation will require significant effort and collaboration. We believe the dialogue emerging from *The Healthcare Imperative* begins to define the opportunities and options for successfully tackling this challenge, and look forward to continued learning from its insights.

Denis A. Cortese
Chair, Roundtable on Value & Science-Driven Health Care

J. Michael McGinnis
Executive Director, Roundtable on Value & Science-Driven Health Care

Arnold Milstein
Planning Committee Chair

Contents

**The contents of the entire report, from
which this Summary is extracted,
are listed below.**

SECTION I: EXCESSIVE HEALTHCARE COSTS

SECTION II: STRATEGIES THAT WORK

SECTION IV: GETTING TO 10 PERCENT

APPENDIXES*

---

*Appendixes A-D are not printed in this book. They are available online at http://www.nap.edu/catalog.php?record_id=12750.

Synopsis and Overview

Framing synopsis. Healthcare cost increases continue to outpace the price and spending growth rates for the rest of the economy by a considerable margin (Bureau of Labor Statistics, 2009). At $2.5 trillion and 17 percent of the nation's gross domestic product in 2009 (CMS, 2009), health spending in the United States commanded twice the per capita expenditures of the average for other developed nations, and concerns have never been higher on the economic implications for individuals, families, businesses, and even the overall capacity and fiscal integrity of critical functions for government at the federal, state, and local levels (Kaiser Family Foundation, 2009a; National Association of State Budget Officers, 2009; Orszag, 2007; Peterson and Burton, 2008).

Moreover, there are compelling signals that much of health spending does little to improve health, and, in certain circumstances, may be associated with poorer health outcomes. Between 2000 and 2006, for example, Medicare spending on imaging services more than doubled, with an over 25 percent increase in use of advanced imaging modalities such as nuclear medicine and CT scans compared to an 18 percent increase in readily available standard imaging modalities such as X-rays and ultrasounds, despite the increased risks associated with advanced imaging services (GAO, 2008). Several recent assessments of institutional and regional variation in costs and volume of treatment services indicate that, in many cases, care profiles that are 60 percent more expensive have no quality advantage (Fisher et al., 2003). Medicare spending per capita by hospital referral region, for example, varied more than threefold—from $5,000 to over $16,000—yet there appeared to be an inverse relationship between healthcare spending and quality scores.

In the face of these urgent challenges, the Institute of Medicine (IOM)—with the support and encouragement of the Peter G. Peterson Foundation—convened four meetings throughout 2009, under the umbrella theme *The Healthcare Imperative: Lowering Costs and Improving Outcomes*. These meetings explored in detail the nature of excess health costs, current evidence on the effectiveness of approaches to their control, the primary opportunities for improvement in the near- and long-terms, and the policy levers necessary to engage. The motivating proposition for the series of meetings was *to reduce healthcare costs by 10 percent within 10 years without compromising patient safety, health outcomes, or valued innovation.* Leading experts from across the nation presented papers and participated in the discussions reflected in this summary publication. The ideas encapsulated throughout this summary reflect only the presentations, discussions, and suggestions that coursed throughout the workshops and should not be construed as consensus or recommendations on specific numbers or actions.

As defined in the meeting planning and presentations, excess health costs derive from the dynamics at play in six overlapping domains of activity.

- Unnecessary services
- Services inefficiently delivered
- Prices that are too high
- Excess administrative costs
- Missed prevention opportunities
- Medical fraud

Because of the overlaps, the difficulty of measurement, and the subjectivity inherent in estimates made under conditions of scientific uncertainty, precision was elusive for estimates of the total amount of excess in the costs of health care. It was, however, notable that estimated totals from three separate approaches discussed in the workshops—extrapolation from observed geographic variation within the United States, contrasting overall U.S. expenditure levels with those of member countries in the Organisation of Economic Co-operation and Development (OECD), and summing the lower bounds of the various estimates for the six domains considered in the IOM workshops—amounted to approximately $750 billion, $760 billion, and $765 billion, respectively, for excess U.S. healthcare costs in 2009.

As meeting discussions focused on the factors at play that give rise to patterns of unnecessary costs, certain elements were most commonly discussed as prominent drivers, noted below and generally working in a mutually reinforcing fashion.

- Scientific uncertainty
- Perverse economic and practice incentives
- System fragmentation
- Opacity as to cost, quality, and outcomes
- Changes in the population's health status
- Lack of patient engagement in decisions
- Under-investment in population health

Discussions on strategies and policies shown in limited assessments to offer solid prospects for simultaneously lowering costs and improving health outcomes included a number of key levers to address the drivers of excess costs.

- Streamlined and harmonized health insurance regulation
- Administrative simplification and consistency
- Payment redesign to focus incentives on results and value
- Quality and consistency in treatment, with a focus on the medically complex
- Evidence that is timely, independent, and understandable

- Transparency requirements as to cost, quality, and outcomes
- Clinical records that are reliable, sharable, and secure
- Data that are protected, but accessible for continuous learning
- Culture and activities framed by patient perspective
- Medical liability reform
- Prevention at the personal and population levels

These are listed in approximate order of the frequency with which they were discussed and do not necessarily reflect an order of priority. For example, the workshop series focus was primarily on medical treatment, and not on prevention, although the latter was clearly discussed as a major strategy of importance. Similarly, medical fraud was specifically not a focus of these discussions but also clearly important to address. In addition, often mentioned was the fact that, like the drivers, they too are interactive with each other, underscoring the fragility of strategies that are singular in nature.

Certain of the participants, invited to offer insights specific to the challenge of reducing healthcare costs by 10 percent within 10 years, individually identified the approaches below as prime candidates for strategy and policy attention to lower costs while improving outcomes, given what is currently known about both the nature of the problems and the availability of potential solutions.

Care-related costs

- Prevent medical errors
- Prevent avoidable hospital admissions
- Prevent avoidable hospital readmissions
- Improve hospital efficiency
- Decrease costs of episodes of care
- Improve targeting of costly services
- Increase shared decision-making

Administrative costs

- Use common billing and claims forms

Related reforms

- Medical liability reform
- Prevent fraud and abuse

Finally, meeting participants identified a number of possible issues and activities for follow-up attention of the Institute of Medicine and its Roundtable on Value & Science-Driven Health Care (formerly the Roundtable on Evidence-Based Medicine), including: consideration of what a strategic roadmap might look like for action priorities and cooperative engagement by Roundtable members; improving the methodologies for estimating the nature and implications of unnecessary healthcare costs; assessing the approaches and potential impact of greater transparency as to healthcare costs, outcomes, and value; and strategies and approaches for providing better perspective to the public on the nature and potential impact of measures to lower costs and improve outcomes of health care in the United States.

National health expenditures are projected to be about $2.5 trillion in 2009, and with growth highly likely to continue to surpass rates for inflation (CMS, 2009), the economic consequences grow increasingly serious for individuals, families, and businesses, as well as states and the federal government. While the consumer price index—a measure estimating the average price of consumer goods and services purchased by households in the United States—*decreased* by 1.5 percent between August 2008 and August 2009, prices for medical services *increased* by 3.3 percent over the same time period (Bureau of Labor Statistics, 2009). As concerns have increased amidst an economic recession, a dominant theme in the health reform dialogue has been the need to control healthcare spending.

It was in this context that the Institute of Medicine's (IOM's) Roundtable on Value & Science-Driven Health Care (formerly the Roundtable on Evidence-Based Medicine), with the support of the Peter G. Peterson Foundation, hosted the four-part series *The Healthcare Imperative: Lowering Costs and Improving Outcomes*. This Summary presents the insights and perspectives arising during the workshop discussions, which explored the drivers of spending, the promising methods of cost control, and the opportunities and barriers to implementing policies. *The motivating goal of the series was to identify ways to reduce healthcare spending by 10 percent from projected expenditures in the United States within the next decade—without compromising health status, quality of care, or valued innovation.*

Part of the National Academies, the IOM has served as the congressionally chartered adviser to the nation on matters of health and health care since its establishment in 1970. With a dedicated commitment to improving the quality of care delivered in the United States, the IOM has conducted a number of highly influential studies—such as *To Err Is Human* (IOM, 2000), *Crossing the Quality Chasm: A New Health System for the 21st Century* (IOM, 2001), and *Rewarding Provider Performance: Aligning Incentives in Medicare* (IOM, 2007)—which have drawn attention to key shortfalls in the performance of the healthcare system, led to demonstrable changes in policy, and helped identify priorities for improving the delivery system.

Similarly, the Peter G. Peterson Foundation acts as an independent, nonpartisan convener and facilitator devoted to the mission of increasing public awareness of the nature and urgency of key economic challenges threatening the nation's fiscal future, and accelerating action by identifying sensible, sustainable solutions. Engaging the range of issues—from debts and deficits to excessive energy consumption and a lagging educational system—threatening the nation's financial future, the Peterson Foundation has committed significant resources and attention to the area of healthcare costs and solutions given health care's direct impact on the economy, including their support for this workshop series.

THE BURDEN OF RISING COST

With projected expenditures of $4.4 trillion in 2018, national health spending could potentially grow more than 300 percent over the course of just 18 years (CMS, 2009). According to projections from the Congressional Budget Office (CBO), federal spending on Medicare and Medicaid alone will increase from about 5 percent of gross domestic product (GDP) in 2009 to more than 6 percent in 2019 and approximately 12 percent by 2050, mostly from growth in per capita costs (Elmendorf, 2009b). If healthcare costs grow at just 2.5 percent more than GDP per capita, by 2050 Medicare and Medicaid expenditures will account for nearly a quarter of the entire U.S. economy (Orszag, 2007).

The costs of health care have therefore not just strained the federal budget; they have affected state governments and the private sector as well. In 2008, Medicaid spending accounted for approximately 21 percent of total state spending and represented the single largest component of state spending (National Association of State Budget Officers, 2009). These levels of healthcare expenditures have restricted the ability of state and local governments to fund other priorities, most prominently the needed investments in education (The White House, 2009).

In the private sector, healthcare costs have contributed to slowing the growth in wages and jobs (National Coalition on Health Care, 2008). While health insurance prices rapidly escalated and employers cut back on the provision of health insurance benefits (Kaiser Family Foundation, 2009b), the number of uninsured rose from 45.7 million in 2007 to 46.3 million in 2008 (U.S. Census Bureau, 2009).

On the individual level, the average cost of annual health insurance premiums for a family of four exceeded $13,000 in 2009, growing five percent in just a single year (Kaiser Family Foundation, 2009a). Health insurance premium increases have consistently exceeded inflation and the growth in worker's wages, forcing individuals to spend increasing amounts of their income simply to maintain health coverage (Kaiser Family Foundation, 2009b). Estimates of the real increase in per capita income devoted to health spending over the next 8 decades have been calculated to be almost 120 percent (Chernew et al., 2009). Fifty-three percent of Americans said their family limited their medical care in the past 12 months because of cost concerns, 19 percent reported serious financial problems due to medical bills, with 13 percent depleting all or most of their savings and 7 percent unable to pay for basic necessities such as food, heat, or housing (Kaiser Family Foundation, 2009c).

While the United States has the highest per capita spending on health care of any industrialized nation—50 percent greater than the second highest and twice as high as the average for Europe (Peterson and Burton, 2008), it continually lags behind other nations on many healthcare outcomes, including life expectancy and infant mortality (Anderson and Frogner, 2008; Docteur and Berenson, 2009). Employers and employees in other industrialized countries spend about 63 percent of what the United States spends on health care, but U.S. workforce health trails by about 10 percent. Indeed, the emerging economies of Brazil, India, and China rank behind the United States by about 5 percent on workforce health measures, but these countries spend only a fraction—about 15 percent—of what the United States spends on health care (Milstein, 2009). The relatively poor performance in health outcomes relative to investment suggests ample opportunity for improvement on both costs and outcomes. This prospect is supported by findings that high spending areas in the United States—spending $6,304 per capita compared to $3,922 per capita in the lowest spending quintile in 1996—utilize sixty percent more frequent physician and hospital visits, testing, and use of procedures yet achieve no quality advantage (Fisher et al., 2003). Together, these findings underscore the opportunities to lower costs without impacting clinical outcomes.

About the Discussion Series

To explore the issues and opportunities central to lowering healthcare expenditures in the United States, the IOM Roundtable on Value & Science-Driven Health Care convened the four-part series *The Healthcare Imperative: Lowering Costs and Improving Outcomes* in May, July, September, and December of 2009 at the National Academies in Washington, DC. These meetings were part of the Roundtable's *Learning Health System* series. The series aimed to gather stakeholders in a trusted venue to engage the issues and concerns needed to facilitate the development of a healthcare system that not only delivers best practices and adds value with each clinical encounter, but adds seamlessly to the knowledge base for health improvement. Motivated by the proposition noted above of reducing per capita health spending in the country by 10 percent within 10 years without compromising health status, quality of care, or innovation, the meeting objectives included: characterizing and discussing the major causes of excess healthcare spending, waste, and inefficiency in the United States; considering the strategies that might reduce per capita health spending in the United States while improving health outcomes; and exploring policy options relevant to those strategies.

With the guidance of a planning committee consisting of leaders representing the various healthcare stakeholders, four meetings were organized:

- The first workshop, titled *Understanding the Targets* and convened on May 21-22, explored the major drivers of healthcare spending growth, focusing on five broad categories: unnecessary services; inefficiently delivered services; excess administrative costs; prices that are too high; and missed prevention opportunities.

- The second workshop, titled *Strategies That Work* and held on July 16-17, focused on the potential of various strategies to lower healthcare spending while improving outcomes, including knowledge enhancement-based strategies; care culture and system redesign-based strategies; transparency of cost and performance; payment and payer-based strategies; community-based and transitional care strategies; and entrepreneurial strategies and potential changes in the state of play.
- The third workshop in the series, titled *The Policy Agenda* and held on September 9-10, explored the policy options to speed adoption of previously discussed strategies to control the drivers of healthcare spending.
- The final meeting in the series, titled *Getting to 10 percent: Opportunities and Requirements* and held on December 15-16, explored in greater detail the priority elements and strategies key to achieving 10 percent savings in healthcare expenditures within 10 years, without compromising health status, quality of care, or valued innovation.

In addition, a commissioned paper was made available as a resource for discussion at the third workshop. This paper placed the preliminary cost estimates offered by presenters at the first two workshops in the context of additional national estimates in the literature. The commissioned paper along with an accompanying summary table, workshop agendas, planning committee and speaker biosketches, and listing of participants are included as appendixes to this publication.

COMMON THEMES

As might be expected for a meeting series exploring—somewhat uniquely—the full range of issues as complex as those involved in understanding and engaging the nature of excessive health costs, discussions throughout the meeting were rich, informative, enlightening, provocative, and, in some cases, even startling. Workshops are explicitly designed to highlight the views of individual participants, and not to seek consensus. Such is certainly the case with the structure of the presentations and discussions in *The Healthcare Imperative: Lowering Costs and Improving Outcomes*. Nonetheless, a number of oft-mentioned—and general—recurring themes coursed throughout the discussion, noted in Box S-1 and summarized below, related to the broad challenges, drivers, and possible levers.

BOX S-1
Common Themes

Cost and outcome challenges

- Health cost excesses with personal, institutional, and national consequences
- Health outcomes far short of expectations
- Fragmented decision points, inconsistent principles, political distortions

Drivers of the shortfalls

- Scientific uncertainty
- Perverse economic and practice incentives
- System fragmentation
- Opacity as to cost, quality, and outcomes
- Changes in the population's health status
- Lack of patient engagement in decisions
- Under-investment in population health

Levers to address the drivers

- Streamlined and harmonized health insurance regulation
- Administrative simplification and consistency
- Payment redesign to focus incentives on results and value
- Quality and consistency in treatment, with a focus on the medically complex
- Evidence that is timely, independent, and understandable
- Transparency requirements as to cost, quality, and outcomes
- Clinical records that are reliable, sharable, and secure
- Data that are protected, but accessible for continuous learning
- Culture and activities framed by patient perspective
- Medical liability reform
- Prevention at the personal and population levels

The Challenges

Health Cost Excesses with Personal, Institutional, and National Consequences

Discussions underscored the expense of our country's healthcare spending both quantitatively and qualitatively. Peter R. Orszag, in his keynote address in *Understanding the Targets*, explained that federal spending on Medicare and Medicaid would grow to unprecedented levels over the coming decades if cost growth continued at uncontrolled levels. He highlighted that Medicare spending per capita by hospital referral region varied more than threefold—from $5,000 to over $16,000—and that this very substantial variation in cost per beneficiary in Medicare is not correlated with overall health outcomes—and, in fact, that the opposite may be the case. Describing the relationship between growing healthcare costs and other sectors of the economy, he also discussed how increasing demands placed on states by Medicaid costs have crowded out other state priorities and limited growth in state appropriations for public education, putting, for example, public universities at risk and at clear competitive disadvantage with their private counterparts in faculty recruitment.

Health Outcomes Far Short of Expectations

Several participants also identified and underscored that not only do our high expenditure levels have a negative impact on families' household budgets and personal health, but the significant variation in care intensity (and expenditures) occurring across the country does not yield notably different outcomes. Indeed, some of the facilities with the best outcomes have lower costs. Often noted was that despite our spending patterns, clinical outcomes, such as life expectancy at birth and care for chronic disease, fall behind in comparison to other countries. Racial disparities in access lead to poorer outcomes, lost productivity, and lower quality of life, which, when compared to groups with the best health outcomes, cost the United States an estimated $229 billion between 2003 and 2006 in direct and indirect medical costs and in the costs of premature death (Laveist et al., 2009). While portions of the population are able to navigate and obtain care almost on demand, others need to rely on the safety net of emergency rooms for the entirety of their care. Even for the insured, the costs of care, geographical impracticalities, and cultural barriers hinder access to care (Devoe et al., 2007; Ngo-Metzger et al., 2003).

Fragmented Decision Points, Inconsistent Principles, Political Distortions

Clear from the discussions was the multifaceted nature of the problem, ranging from poor care coordination, lack of consistent evidence-based guidelines, and medical errors resulting from multiple handoffs, to inconsistencies in the policies of health insurance regulators, payment systems that encourage volume over value, and political influences that sometimes overturn scientific determinations. The clearest common denominator is the level of fragmentation in key system decision points, which challenges both the timely marshaling of evidence for decisions and consistency of its application. While almost two-thirds of consumers believe that their care is already evidence-based (Brownlee, 2009), many participants identified the lack of consistency with which evidence-based medicine is truly practiced. Individual attendees cited inconsistent guideline application as leading to variations in clinical decisions and practice patterns. To address the interests of the various stakeholders in health care, who frequently fail to harmonize in the best interests of patients, attendees asserted the need for multipronged solutions. Suggestions to effectively address the root causes of spending growth in the nation ranged from regulatory policy reform to provider and consumer-based initiatives.

The Drivers

Discussions identified a number of factors driving expenditure growth, noting several in particular.

Scientific Uncertainty

Many participants remarked that the development of clinical evidence needed significant investments, given the continuous emergence of new therapies, pharmaceuticals, and technologies. Despite the work of various medical and scientific organizations, the gap between practice needs and available guidance was described as growing. An additional level of near-term complexity was introduced by emerging insights from the field of genomics (Farnham, 2009; U.S. Department of Energy Biological and Environmental Research Program, 2009). Discoveries about genetic variation clearly increase the amount of information needed to properly target diagnostic and therapeutic interventions. When tools are available to appropriately triage insights from research into application for targeting, care should eventually become much more specific and effective (Pollack, 2008).

Perverse Economic and Practice Incentives

Various attendees cited the current, predominantly fee-for-service reimbursement system as providing perverse incentives, rewarding volume of services over the delivery of high-value services. Citing the variable rates of back surgeries, invasive cardiac interventions, and rates of specialist consultations between hospitals, states, and regions that yielded no discernible quality differences (Delaune and Everett, 2008), many participants discussed the need to shift the focus to patient-centered value. Compounding the problem of economic incentives promoting volume over value, the implicit pressures of the medical liability environment and defensive medicine were noted as contributing substantially to the delivery of unnecessary services. Much higher reimbursement levels for specialty over primary care further distort the incentives for certain services.

System Fragmentation

Discussions highlighted the pervasive fragmentation of the health-care system on virtually every dimension—providers, payers, regulators, consumers—as a fundamental challenge to efficient and effective care. Fragmented communication between providers, duplicative testing and the absence of vital information compromise both outcomes and economic prospects—discontinuities that pose costs to both patients and society (Valenstein and Schifman, 1996). While patients were described as having to complete paperwork requesting the same information again and again, providers were also identified as suffering from a lack of harmonization around administrative policies and reporting requirements from payers and quality monitors. Information needed for provider credentialing was requested repeatedly by differing institutions, consuming time and resources that could otherwise be spent on patient care (Healthcare Administration Simplification Coalition, 2009).

Opacity as to Cost, Quality, and Outcomes

Without meaningful and trustworthy sources of information on health-care costs, quality, outcomes, and value, patients were described as becoming disempowered in the decision-making process. One participant likened being a patient in the healthcare system to being a tourist in a foreign country without knowledge of the language, geography, or customs (Rein, 2007). Similarly, without reliable, publicly available information on resource use and quality, providers were identified in several discussions as lacking either an understanding of their performance relative to their peers or an impetus to improve the value of the care they deliver. Many proposed that current approaches to improving health care in the United States are grounded in market forces, but those forces cannot work properly until consumers have better information about the nature and value of the elements.

Changes in the Population's Health Status

Since 48 percent of Medicare beneficiaries have at least three chronic conditions and 21 percent have five or more conditions, it has been estimated that approximately 60 million Americans have multiple morbidities, a number that is expected to increase to 81 million by 2020 (Anderson and Horvath, 2002). Additionally, projections place levels of obesity at 41 percent by 2015 (Wang and Beydoun, 2007), with consequences for diabetes, heart disease, hypertension, cancer, and osteoarthritis. In conjunction with an aging population, several attendees suggested that the changing demography of the nation's health precipitated the need to increase prevention efforts, lower the prevalence of obesity, and facilitate management of multiple co-occurring and increasingly complex chronic conditions.

Lack of Patient Engagement in Decisions

Several conversations identified patient engagement as a critical element of treatment success but emphasized that consumers may be the least informed on issues related to costs, outcomes, or value. Almost 40 percent of Americans possess only "basic" or "below-basic" health literacy skills (Kutner et al., 2006). With patients' already limited understanding of health information, their ability to engage in informed decision making becomes increasingly insufficient as the volume and complexity of data available to them increases (Greene et al., 2008). In addition, the amount of information available to patients on the Internet holds the prospect of equipping patients to be active partners with clinicians in their care, but it was suggested by some that professional culture lags behind the potential in this respect.

Under-Investment in Population Health

Given the significant dependence of health status on the dynamics of physical, behavioral, and social determinants (WHO, 2009), full attainment of each individual's health potential requires strong commitments, investment, and progress in population-wide health programs (e.g., public health and health promotion-related activities), suggested many discussants. Estimates suggest that the potential to improve the health of a group is far less a matter of the health care received than of members' experience in the other domains of health determinants. Yet the dialogue called attention to the fact that only about 6 percent of national health expenditures is spent on public and population health (CMS, 2009). Several participants identified the critical role that prevention and population health—which broadly encompasses health outcomes and their biomedical and social determinants (Kindig and Stoddart, 2003)—could play in lowering the burden of chronic illness and improving productivity and quality of life.

The Levers

Attendees spoke broadly of the key levers for catalyzing transformation of the delivery system.

Streamlined and Harmonized Health Insurance Regulation

Many participants posited that addressing system fragmentation required effective streamlining of the diverse protocols and requirements arising from interactions between insurance companies, myriad employers and provider organizations, 51 state insurance commissions, and public payers. Streamlining techniques intended to foster simplification through regional approaches and national guidelines and standards have had burgeoning success with public–private partnerships but still have underrealized potential (Healthcare Administration Simplification Coalition, 2009; IBM Global Business Services, 2009).

Administrative Simplification and Consistency

Physicians spend a reported 43 minutes per day on average—the equivalent of 3 hours per week and nearly 3 weeks per year—on administrative interactions with health plans and not on patient care (Casalino et al., 2009). It was also noted that one assessment found surgical nurses spending about a third of their time on documentation needs rather than clinical care (Smith, 2009). Many participants characterized efforts to streamline and harmonize payment and reporting requirements as basic, straightforward, and practical prerequisites to eliminating substantial systemic administrative costs.

Payment Redesign to Focus Incentives on Results and Value

Based on encouraging signs from demonstrations and theoretical models, many attendees suggested that much may be gained (lower costs, better outcomes) from broad changes to focus payments on episodes, outcomes, and value and to better target resources to those patients at highest risk of poor outcomes. Consideration of a proposed Independent Medicare Advisory Council to issue recommendations for Medicare payment updates and broader reforms that would not increase the aggregate level of net Medicare expenditures (Orszag, 2009) was discussed as a possibility, as were incentives for team care, provider integration, and patient involvement.

Quality and Consistency in Treatment, with a Focus on the Medically Complex

With more than 3,000 guidelines from more than 280 organizations registered with the National Guideline Clearinghouse (2009), consistency in guideline recommendations was raised as a concern. Also discussed was the need for a trusted means to broker differences in recommendations and channel them into effective use. It was also noted by many that with a dedicated commitment to effectiveness studies embedded in the notion of a *learning health system* and additional measures that allowed capture of effectiveness data directly from the care process, significant insights could emerge to provide greater consistency in guideline development.

Evidence That Is Timely, Independent, and Understandable

To improve and reinforce evidence on effective care, several exchanges highlighted the need for a dedicated, unified program to fill the substantial gaps in reliable guidance, keep up with innovation and the changing science, and improve practice reliability, consistency, and impact. Mandated by the American Recovery and Reinvestment Act (ARRA) of 2009, the IOM recently recommended a priority list of the 100 top investigative topics for comparative effectiveness research (CER). Simultaneously, the newly formed Federal Coordinating Council for Comparative Effectiveness Research provided recommendations on infrastructure and organizational expenditures for CER within the federal government. In concert with the $1.1 billion appropriated to the Department of Health and Human Services for CER, various attendees voiced hope that action on these recommendations and the resulting CER research findings would guide future treatment decisions, reimbursement structures, and benefit designs by placing greater emphasis on value.

Transparency Requirements as to Cost, Quality, and Outcomes

With price and quality transparency viewed as critical elements of a consumerism strategy (Tynan et al., 2008), many participants identified pairing the development of information in accessible formats regarding cost, outcomes, and value with governance and administrative streamlining as having the potential to accelerate focus on value's key ingredients. Increasing access to practical, usable transparency information could marshal patient and consumer involvement in improving the value of care. Some participants noted a 38 percent increase in information-seeking behaviors related to health in 6 years. In 2007, for example, 56 percent of American adults—more than 122 million people—sought information about a personal health concern, with particularly notable increases in use of the Internet as a source of health information (Hu and Cohen, 2008).

Clinical Records That Are Reliable, Sharable, and Secure

Use of electronic health records was noted throughout the discussions, not as a panacea, but as a tool to enhance the effectiveness and efficiency of medical care, facilitate patient handoffs, provide decision prompts at the point of choice, and strengthen patient involvement in the care process. The attention and resources dedicated to health information technology in recent legislation reflect the significant potential for electronic health records (EHRs) to facilitate care coordination and minimize medical errors (CBO,

2008b). Discussions underscored the need to facilitate the technical aspects of adoption and utilization while simultaneously expanding the research capacity of EHRs.

Data That Are Protected But Accessible for Continuous Learning

With more than 30 billion healthcare transactions occurring verbally, on paper, and electronically each year (Menduno, 1999), participants discussed the concept of harnessing the power of information generated from current clinical care. Many suggested that not only might electronic records improve clinical decision making and handoffs, but clinical data should be considered a knowledge utility. As a resource for real-time monitoring of the results of treatment and ongoing generation of new evidence for effective care, several individuals suggested that electronic health records have the ability to facilitate continuous improvement in the quality of care delivered.

Culture and Activities Framed by Patient Perspective

With 25 percent of Medicare expenditures attributed to unwanted variation in preference-sensitive care (Wennberg, 2008), it was noted by many participants that much of healthcare delivery has been shaped over the past generation with the primary convenience and interests of the clinician, not the patient, in mind. Yet, not only for patient satisfaction, but for better patient outcomes, attendees noted that the lens has to focus on patient perspectives and needs. Several participants suggested that shared decision making utilizing patient-centric decision aids have been demonstrated not only to facilitate patient engagement and understanding but also to ensure that the personal preferences of patients are reflected in the ultimate treatment choice.

Medical Liability Reform

While the number of medical malpractice payments reached almost 16,000 in 2006 with mean payments to plaintiffs of approximately $312,000 (National Practitioner Data Bank, 2006), malpractice premiums have continued to increase relentlessly, in some states by up to 73 percent in 2002 (Thorpe, 2004). Because defensive medicine appears to be a significant driver of unnecessary services, many participants referenced reforms—such as the notion of a "safe harbor" for best evidence practices, caps on noneconomic damages, and specialized tribunals—as important to reducing costs.

Prevention at the Personal and Population Levels

Many discussants often referred to the cost, now and in the future, of obesity among Americans, which if unchecked might lead to Medicare expenditures that are a third higher for obese patients than for those of normal weight (Lakdawalla et al., 2005). They also spoke of the burdens of chronic conditions, whose treatment consumes 96 cents per dollar for Medicare and 83 cents per dollar for Medicaid (Partnership to Fight Chronic Disease, 2009). While discussing possible solutions ranging from clinical preventive services to community health, several participants suggested that the distinctions between wellness, prevention, and treatment of chronic diseases were artificial because all were essential and required strong community initiative.

Because the discussion series took place during a period of active focus and debate related to health reform, the discussion during the third meeting, which was devoted to drawing from insights of prior presentations, was particularly helpful in offering framing considerations of the broad implications for reform. Participants at that meeting variously articulated a number of observations providing a constructive context for considering the common themes noted above, as well as the individual summaries in the chapters that follow. They include issues related to reorientation to patient-centered value; payment reform; multimodality of approach; specificity of responsibilities; incrementalism; transparency and accountability; and collaboration.

WORKSHOP ONE: UNDERSTANDING THE TARGETS

The first workshop, titled Understanding the Targets explored the major drivers of excess spending in health care, focusing on the categories below:

- Unnecessary services;
- Inefficiently delivered medical services;
- Excess administrative costs;
- Prices that are too high; and
- Missed prevention opportunities

As noted earlier, Office of Management and Budget Director Orszag led off the workshop and the series with a keynote address that emphasized the compelling challenges to the nation's fiscal integrity, focusing on the growth of health costs and individual and societal consequences. He underscored the importance of understanding, engaging, and controlling the waste and excess that were the focus of the workshop framework.

Within this framework, presenters provided qualitative descriptions of the nature of the issue and its most important elements, quantitative dollar estimates of the respective contribution to overall unnecessary health costs, and a sense of the relative importance of the major contributors within the category. Given the complexity of the issues, participants also identified further issues for refinement in order to maximize the accuracy and completeness of the calculations, including additional accounting for overlaps between areas to minimize double-counting and the multifaceted nature of the issues discussed, such as the relative impacts and differences among commercially- and publicly-insured beneficiaries. For example, there are areas of overlap and interaction between the costs of uncoordinated care and the overuse of discretionary services that are difficult to disentangle. It was clear from the presentations that no single issue dominates healthcare spending growth, and that it is the result of multiple forces at play in a fragmented delivery system. Below brief summaries of the individual presentations are presented.

Unnecessary Services

Speakers in this session examined the provision of unnecessary services, highlighting the consequences of scientific uncertainty, perverse economic and practice incentives, and lack of patient engagement in decisions (Chapter 2).

Cost of Overuse: Services Provided Beyond Evidence-Established Levels

Amitabh Chandra examined the relationship between mortality and spending in hospitals. Using mortality as a quality measure and Medicare spending per beneficiary as the expenditure measure, he explained that if lower performing hospitals could be made to perform like higher performing ones, this would result in 8 percent reductions in both cost and mortality for three high-mortality conditions (acute myocardial infarction, hip fracture, and colon cancer). This is the equivalent of over $1 billion annually and over 11,500 patients receiving at least one more year of life. While this analysis was limited by the author's ability to adequately risk-adjust claims data, it was suggested that with savings of this magnitude for just three conditions, the potential across all conditions and populations could be substantial. Chandra concluded that these findings support a broader message that, despite the inefficiencies within the American healthcare system, it is possible to save both money and lives.

Cost of Discretionary Use Beyond Benchmarks

Focusing on services for which evidence indicated are unjustified, Elliott S. Fisher discussed the considerable regional variation in both practice and spending occurring across the nation, identifying the over-utilization of discretionary services as a main contributing factor. Such services included more frequent visits to physicians, greater use of the hospital as a site of care, and greater use of imaging, diagnostic tests, and minor procedures. Using the lowest spending regions as benchmarks to estimate the magnitude of potential savings that could be achieved within the U.S. healthcare system, his analyses suggested that hospital utilization could decline by between 23 percent and 28 percent, primary care visits by 12 percent to 16 percent and medical specialist visits by 37 percent to 44 percent. Fisher acknowledged that this analysis was based solely on Medicare data and did not account for the significant variation that occurs within regions, but he estimated that should all spending regions achieve the benchmarks set by the lowest spending regions, savings to the Medicare program alone could total 18 percent to 20 percent of current spending, or $48 billion to $54 billion per year. Therefore, Fisher suggested, a gradual transition toward a more frugal healthcare system is not only possible, but it could in his view yield substantial savings without lowering quality.

Cost of Unnecessary Choice of Higher Cost Services

David Wennberg discussed the large variation in preference sensitive care—which accounts for 25 percent of all Medicare expenditures—and how this may be rooted in frequent encouragement to have physicians drive medical decision making rather than actively sharing the decision-making process with patients. He reviewed evidence that shared decision making (SDM) with decision aids provided an effective tool to ensure that the personal values and preferences of patients were reflected in the ultimate treatment selection. Extrapolating from studies demonstrating the impact of SDM—such as a reduction in surgical procedures by 25 percent compared to usual care—he calculated that systematic use of shared decision making coupled with provider incentives and changes in benefit design could reduce unwarranted variation in service utilization and yield up to 5 percent in net savings, the equivalent of $125 billion in 2009. Wennberg cautioned that data was still needed to assess the financial impact of provider-based SDM on total expenditures, and the effect benefit designs and reimbursement models could have on increasing use of SDM. However, given the potential savings, he recommended a paradigm shift from informed patient consent to informed patient choice.

Inefficiently Delivered Services

The presenters in this session focused on the savings opportunities available if appropriate services were provided in the most efficient ways possible, drawing clear connections to the problems resulting from underlying system fragmentation, and perverse economic and practice incentives (Chapter 3).

Cost of Mistakes (Medical Errors, Preventable Complications)

Ashish Jha focused on the challenges of medical errors and duplicative testing in U.S. hospitals. Using a comprehensive literature review to identify rates of adverse events and redundant tests in hospitals and data from the National Inpatient Sample, he determined that over 3 million preventable adverse events occur in hospitals annually, with over half of these due to hospital-acquired infections and adverse drug events. He estimated that, in 2004 alone, eliminating readily preventable adverse events would result in direct savings of over $16 billion (6 percent of total inpatient costs) while eliminating redundant tests would save an additional $8 billion (3 percent of total inpatient costs). In describing the limitations of his analysis, he highlighted in particular that the estimates were based on data that were several years old, and therefore may not reflect current costs, and that data were not available for all patient populations (e.g., women admitted to the hospital for labor and delivery). Jha concluded by suggesting that improving quality of care while saving costs will require additional efforts to systematically measure and publicly report adverse event rates in U.S. hospitals.

Cost of Unnecessary Use of Higher Cost Providers

Considering the significant operating expenses due to the costs of medical labor, Gary S. Kaplan suggested that efficient use of skilled mid-level providers could reduce healthcare costs substantially for both purchasers and providers. Using the care pathway for breast nodules as an example, he explained that more than 90 percent of patients with breast nodules do not require surgery. Using an experienced Advanced Registered Nurse Practitioner (ARNP) instead of a breast surgeon for the initial office visit could reduce the cost of providing care. In the back pain care pathway, substituting an initial physician evaluation with an initial evaluation performed by a physical therapist with minimal physician support could achieve similar savings while simultaneously improving access, patient satisfaction, and the patient's return to function. Based on his experience that ARNP or Physician Assistant providers could deliver at least 50 percent of episodes of care for uncomplicated medical conditions, he surmised that use of mid-level practitioners rather than physicians could save an additional $8 billion in annual spending. In closing, he outlined key factors to affordable health care, including: accountability; efficient use of labor; use of effective care pathways for high-cost conditions; alignment of reimbursement with value; and electronic health records embedded with evidence-based decision rules.

Cost of Operational Inefficiencies at Care Delivery Sites

Focusing on waste occurring within medical practices as a consequence of inefficient clinical and administrative processes, William F. Jessee drew upon a variety of data collected by the Medical Group Management Association (MGMA) from medical groups throughout the United States to estimate the savings potentially realizable from improving efficiency in physician offices. He offered that savings from efficiency and streamlining might approximate $6 billion annually, about 0.2 percent of total healthcare costs in the United States. While Jessee suggested that this estimate was provocative, he also cautioned that it was preliminary in nature, as it was based on limited cross-sectional survey data. Focusing on inefficiencies in hospitals, Arnold Milstein described analyses of the Medicare Payment Advisory Commission to identify hospitals ranked in the top 12 percent on a composite measure of low risk-adjusted cost per case and high quality scores. He suggested that, if the other 88 percent of U.S. hospitals replicated their attainment, their 30 day mortality could decline by 18 percent, readmissions by 4 percent, and inpatient costs by 12 percent while patients' experiences would be unaffected. This would result in an average reduction in U.S. hospital inpatient cost per case of approximately 11 percent. If these hospital cost savings were passed along to consumers, it would lower U.S. healthcare spending by approximately 2 percent. Milstein suggested that the most promising approach to reaping the savings appears to be the combination of dissemination of standardized care pathways and other successful elements of clinical process reengineering in top-performing hospitals with more pro-competitive health industry regulatory policies.

Cost of Care Fragmentation

Mary Kay Owens subsequently explored the impact of uncoordinated and fragmented health care on patients. In a review of utilization and expenditures for medical services and drugs (which included a detailed assessment of the costs of avoidable emergency department visits, duplicative and unnecessary drugs, and other types of medical services), she identified significant trends among those Medicaid patients receiving uncoordinated care. They represented less than 10 percent of patients but accounted for an average of 46 percent of drug costs, 32 percent of medical costs, and 36 percent of total costs for the population. Extrapolating to the publicly and privately insured, she calculated that, with a multiple intervention approach designed to identify patients with the most extreme uncoordinated care and facilitate their care coordination, annual savings of $271 billion could accrue nationally by 2014. Owens emphasized that these estimates do not account for the population of uninsured, nor do they factor in future demographic trends in chronic disease or a growing elderly population.

Excess Administrative Costs

The presenters in this session approached estimating excess administrative costs from a variety of macro- and microeconomic levels, all with the goal of identifying the portion of expenditures spent on administration that could be reduced by increasing the efficiency of the delivery system, which highlighted the need for administrative simplification and harmonization (Chapter 4).

Insurance Administrative Costs Beyond Benchmarks

James G. Kahn identified a major portion of administrative costs as due to billing and insurance-related (BIR) activities undertaken to fulfill the requirements of getting paid, from contracting through collections. Building on this idea, and as noted earlier, Lawrence P. Casalino described how physicians spend the equivalent of 3 hours per week and nearly 3 weeks per year just on administrative interactions with health plans, and not on patient care. This is the equivalent of $31 billion in costs to practices, much of which is excess.

Drawing on existing research, Kahn and the other presenters in this session estimated that the BIR portion of physician revenue was estimated at 13 percent, an estimated $70 billion per year. For hospital care, they estimated BIR costs of $67 billion. The total for physicians and hospitals was calculated to be $137 billion per year. If a similar rate applied to other providers (e.g., pharmacies and nursing homes), he estimated the total BIR costs for all providers at approximately $214 billion and the total BIR costs for private insurers at $105 billion and for public programs at $42 billion. Adding each of the individual BIR estimates together, they suggested a total upper bound for BIR costs of $361 billion in 2009. However, they also encouraged caution in interpreting the results given the lack of adequate data on the BIR costs in several settings, such as in pharmacies and nursing homes.

In addition, Andrew L. Naugle considered reduction of commercial payer administrative expense as an opportunity to generate substantial financial savings for the U.S. healthcare system. For 2008, he identified approximately 11 percent ($42 billion) of total fully-insured commercial health insurance premiums as being consumed by payer administrative activities such as claim processing, customer service, medical management, and sales and marketing, as well as corporate overhead and external broker commissions. If the average payer administrative expense level for fully-insured commercial products were reduced to approximately 8 percent of premiums—an expense level exhibited by "best practice" payers—he suggested that total payer administrative expense for these products would be reduced to approximately $29 billion, thereby generating a savings of approximately $14 billion; for the self-insured market, he estimated an additional savings of $6 billion to $9 billion could be realized. As these estimates applied data across the entire commercial marketplace, Naugle cautioned that variation in savings could occur across specific individual payers as they each will be variously impacted by their respective marketplace and organizational characteristics. Outlining opportunities to capitalize on the potential savings, he discussed possible policy options, including the elimination of manual transactions between payers and providers; simplifying the sales process; maximizing self-service capabilities and adoption; and standardizing payer and provider interaction processes and rules.

Care Site Administrative Costs Beyond Benchmarks

James L. Heffernan described physician billing costs as a substantial component of administrative costs, and comparatively higher than the costs for similar functions in other industries. Modeling the cost of administrative complexity burden of a physicians' organization by comparing the costs of the current system versus a uniform and transparent set of payment rules, he described analyses yielding an estimated administrative burden of 11 percent of net patient service revenue. Extrapolating nationally from the experience of one professional billing office, Heffernan estimated this totals $26 billion, thus suggesting that a single transparent set of payment rules in a multipayer healthcare system would potentially reduce the burdens on a provider's billing office.

Regulatory and Compliance-Imposed Costs Beyond Benchmarks

In his presentation on clinical data knowledge utilities, Peter K. Smith suggested that medical documentation requirements currently result in a vast dataset that is not relevant to patient-specific needs. In addition, he stated that current documentation considers important clinical elements relevant to a patient's specific problem to be secondary to the necessity of supporting payment requirements and ensuring the ability to defend against medical liability. He further described an analysis indicating that surgical nurses spend the greatest proportion of their time (36 percent) on documentation, compared to 19 percent on patient care activities and 21 percent on care coordination. Applying this proportion to the national health expenditure estimates, Smith estimated that nursing documentation costs an estimated $147 billion per year; reducing this documentation by 60 percent could yield $88 billion in savings, representing 4 percent of total national health expenditures. Therefore, Smith expressed the view that the goals of the expansive clinical regulatory requirements may well be misaligned and possibly contrary to effective healthcare delivery.

Prices That Are Too High

The speakers in this session explored how current market practices result from perverse economic and practice incentives, and the opacity of cost, quality, and outcomes, yielding prices that may cost the nation billions of dollars in expenditures unnecessarily (Chapter 5).

Service Prices Beyond Competitive Benchmarks

Cory S. Capps focused on the consequences of hospital consolidations, describing recent trends and evidence from economic and health services research that found that consolidation often results in higher prices for hospital services. Using national data on the system affiliations of hospitals and other hospital characteristics and results from the existing economic literature, he quantified the likely effects of consolidation on the prices paid to hospitals for inpatient care and estimated the contribution of hospital consolidation to overall healthcare spending. Based on this analysis, he suggested that total national healthcare expenditures were roughly 0.4 percent to 0.5 percent higher ($10 billion to $12 billion in annual expenditures) than they would be absent the price increases resulting from hospital consolidation. However, he also explained that this analysis considers only broad averages and general trends, and does not indicate that any specific hospital consolidation will (or will not) result in higher or lower prices.

In addition to hospital services prices, the background material commissioned to inform the workshop series discussion identified analyses on physician pricing indicated that U.S. specialists make 6.5 times per capita GDP, compared with an average of 3.9 times for member countries of the Organisation of Economic Co-operation and Development (OECD) (Farrell et al., 2008). The analyses additionally indicated that, across all U.S. physicians, higher earnings add $64 billion in costs to the U.S. system, the sum of $49 billion more for specialists and $15 billion more for generalists.

Product Prices Beyond Competitive Benchmarks

Pharmaceuticals Jack Hoadley explored the factors involved in the pricing of medications, highlighting that drugs are priced differently across the various segments of the U.S. pharmaceutical market. As an example, he discussed how government-sponsored programs, such as the Department of Veterans Affairs and Medicaid, price drugs differently than privately

insured health plans. He also identified brand name drugs under patent protection as being priced differently than those where multiple manufacturers
compete to sell the product. He also suggested that there are distinctive
approaches for drugs delivered by physicians (e.g., chemotherapy drugs)
or in institutional settings (e.g., hospitals or nursing homes). In looking at
system-wide savings from lower prices, he estimated that a 5 percent reduction in the price of brand drugs across all payers, except those government
payers already obtaining deep discounts, would yield about $9 billion in
annual savings. While Hoadley cautioned that this estimate is only illus-
trative, as no obvious standard for an optimal drug price is available, he
also explained that additional consideration of the impact price alterations
could have on research and development and innovation is necessary.

Durable medical equipment   Thomas J. Hoerger and Mark E. Wynn turned
their attention to the pricing of durable medical equipment (DME), a category of health expenditures that includes oxygen equipment, wheelchairs,
and other equipment and supplies used in the home as well as eyeglasses
and hearing aids. They discussed evidence that equipment prices may be
too high, including data from competitive bidding, which resulted in price
reductions of 20 percent in a Medicare demonstration project from 1998
to 2002. Based on these results, Hoerger estimated a potential savings of
approximately $3 billion, which equaled 28 percent of current Medicare
payments for DME and converted to about 12 percent of the $255 bil-
lion total expenditures on DME and 0.1 percent of the $2 trillion in total
national health expenditures in 2007. Care as to the interpretation of the
amount of savings achievable was suggested by Hoerger because, while
these calculations were based on competitive bidding results from the 1999-
2002 demonstration projects and the 2008 national program, Medicare fees
for DME have since been reduced.

Devices   Jeffrey C. Lerner examined the field of medical devices and technology, exploring how fair prices could be negotiated between buyer and
seller so that waste can be minimized. Based on his analyses, he estimated
that hospitals, the primary purchasers of devices, would have saved approximately 3 percent or $5 billion in 2008 had they negotiated with manufac-
turers to achieve the average savings for every device they bought. He also
acknowledged that beyond hospitals, data from outpatient medical centers
and physician groups would be needed for a more complete analysis.

Missed Prevention Opportunities

These presentations explored how changing demographic trends in
the population's health status and underinvestment in population health

contribute to missed prevention opportunities, and focused not simply on the potential costs of missed prevention opportunities but also on the added value of increasing the delivery of preventive efforts to patients (Chapter 6).

Primary and Secondary Prevention

Steven H. Woolf stressed the consequences of an inadequate emphasis on disease prevention, including greater morbidity and mortality and lower quality-of-life that would occur because of missed opportunities to prevent disease and injury (primary prevention) and from missed opportunities to control or reverse pre-symptomatic disease (secondary prevention). While he emphasized the importance of community- or population-based prevention services, he used obesity as a case study to demonstrate how lost opportunities in prevention result in measurable health costs and excess resource consumption. He concluded by asserting that slowing the growth of healthcare spending will ultimately necessitate redistributing current expenditures to high-value services such as prevention.

Thomas J. Flottemesch described how underutilization of preventive services represented missed opportunities for reducing future medical costs. He presented estimates on the delivery costs and potential medical savings of 20 evidence-based primary and secondary clinical preventive services using 2006 cost and utilization data. While acknowledging that certain costs could have been omitted or double-counted due to insufficient data, he suggested an estimated net medical cost savings of $7 billion or a 0.4 percent reduction in personal healthcare expenditures from increased use of recommended primary preventive services. Conversely, he found that none of the included secondary preventive services were cost saving. Flottemesch concluded that, while different types of evidence-based clinical preventive services have the potential for differential impacts depending upon current delivery rates and target populations, evidence-based preventive services should be embraced, and their use encouraged, because of their positive health impact.

Tertiary Prevention

Michael P. Pignone focused on better use of effective strategies for preventing disease progression and further adverse health events in patients with established health issues (tertiary prevention). Examining the evidence on several specific types of services, including interventions to reduce re-hospitalizations for a range of conditions, disease management interventions for chronic conditions such as heart failure and diabetes, and greater use of effective therapies in patients with known coronary heart disease, he surmised that widespread adoption of proven programs for key chronic conditions could produce substantial national savings, perhaps as much as $45 billion per year. However, he also explained that translating successful interventions to new populations and settings and realizing savings may be difficult because of the differing organizational and population needs of individual institutions and communities. Despite these limitations, he ultimately suggested that better use of effective tertiary prevention possesses strong potential for improving health and reducing spending.

International Context

Focusing on a comparison between U.S. and international trends in healthcare expenditures, this presentation underscored the nature of our system's fragmentation, changing health demographics, and perverse economic and practice incentives (Chapter 1).

Comparison to OECD Countries

Eric Jensen described analyses concluding that the United States spends nearly $650 billion more on health care than one would expect based on the nation's wealth and the experience of other OECD countries. Of this amount, he related that nearly two-thirds or $436 billion is attributable to outpatient care, which is partly due to an ongoing structural shift away from inpatient settings that should in theory reduce total system costs. However, it was estimated that the United States saves at most $100 billion to $120 billion in inpatient care costs as a consequence of our capacity to provide care in an outpatient setting, far less than the $436 billion in above expected costs. In addition to this structural change, several other factors fuel the growth in outpatient care costs, including (1) the highly profitable nature of outpatient care; (2) the judgment-based nature of physician care coupled with the fee-for-service reimbursement; (3) unit price growth linked to technological innovation; (4) demand growth linked to greater availability of supply; and (5) insurance contracts with limited out-of-pocket costs making patients relatively price-insensitive. He also explored factors driving higher than expected costs in other parts of the U.S. healthcare system including the cost of drugs ($98 billion above expected) and health administration and insurance ($91 billion above expected). Offering a framework for reform, he stated that policy makers must address supply and demand, focus on healthcare financing, and institute an effective organizational framework for implementation.

WORKSHOP TWO: STRATEGIES THAT WORK

The second workshop explored the major methods of controlling healthcare spending growth, focusing on six broad categories:

- Knowledge enhancement-based strategies;
- Care culture and system redesign-based strategies;
- Transparency of cost and results;
- Payment and payer-based strategies;
- Community-based and transitional care strategies; and
- Entrepreneurial strategies.

Laying the groundwork for subsequent presentations with his keynote address for the second workshop, titled Strategies That Work, Glenn Steele, Jr., described how Geisinger Health System has leveraged its position as both provider and payer to innovate within the current delivery system without developing new operational and financial problems. He described their pioneering work with bundled payments for cardiac surgery, which has yielded significant improvements in the delivery of evidence-based care and decreased re-hospitalizations within 30 days by 44 percent. With a focus on the high-utilizing chronic disease population, Steele relayed that their care management initiative has reduced readmission rates among the targeted population by nearly 30 percent within a year and decreased total medical costs by 4 percent—a return-on-investment of 250 percent. He also described the positive externalities arising from their innovations, citing how the teachers in Danville, Pennsylvania received an average raise of $7,000 due to Geisinger's ability to decrease health insurance costs. Identifying Geisinger's organization, local marketplace, financial health and planning, and the sociology of its catchment area as key elements of their local environment, he characterized the success of their interventions in acute and chronic care as steeped in their ability to innovate, experiment, and learn "on the fly."

Presentations throughout this workshop provided an overview of the evidence supporting the impacts of the strategy being considered and several offered quantitative dollar estimates of the savings achievable from nationwide implementation. While reflecting on the analytics, participants and a panel of economists including Dana Goldman, Eric Jensen, Len Nichols, Robert D. Reischauer, and Jonathan S. Skinner noted the need to account for possible synergies between strategies, such as the impact of tort reform and health information technology (HIT) with decision support on defensive medicine practices. Similar to the drivers of healthcare cost growth discussed in the first workshop, participants referenced the need for multifaceted strategies in order to effectively bend the cost curve. Brief summaries of the individual presentations are presented below.

Knowledge Enhancement

Speakers in this session focused on the essential strategies to enable more efficient generation and application of knowledge during the care process, in particular highlighting tools for generating high quality, consistent treatment, with a focus on the medically complex; timely, independent, and understandable evidence; reliable, sharable, and secure clinical records; protected but accessible data; and patient-centered care (Chapter 8).

Use of Evidence-Based Clinical Practice Protocols

Lucy A. Savitz drew on experiences from Intermountain Healthcare to demonstrate the potential for evidence-based clinical protocols to improve outcomes and lower costs. She described the advantages of these protocols as: providing readily accessible references to knowledge in guidelines that have been selected for use in a specific clinical context; improving the clarity of an existing guideline; facilitating tailoring of guidelines to a patient's specific clinical state; and providing timely decision support that is specific for the patient. Using the example of a single evidence-based care process model as an example, she suggested that savings seen at Intermountain from implementation and utilization of this model for febrile infants extrapolated nationally would yield an estimated $2 billion savings annually. The system-wide and condition-wide implications, she noted, are clearly considerable if similar reliability and consistency of care could be widely harmonized. While suggesting that Intermountain's protocols could be adopted across different models of care delivery, she additionally discussed the larger challenge of sustainability of savings beyond initial implementation.

Decision Support Provided Through Electronic Health Records

With accumulating evidence that EHRs can improve the efficiency, quality, and safety of health care by providing more complete information with evidence-based decision support to physicians at the point of care, Rainu Kaushal explored the potential of EHRs to lower costs and improve outcomes. She suggested that interoperability and the inclusion of electronic prescribing functionalities are particularly important in generating value, as is extensive technical support to achieve appropriate implementation and use. She reviewed published literature estimating that adoption of nationwide interoperable EHRs could save $77 billion annually. Additional literature estimated that inpatient computer physician order entry (CPOE) adoption could yield savings ranging from $1 million to almost $3 million annually per hospital after an initial investment, and savings from adoption of EHRs in the ambulatory setting were estimated to be $86,400 per provider over 5 years. However, Kaushal underscored that the estimates described were restrained by the limited availability of primary data and consequent heavy reliance on expert estimates. She also suggested that the critical cofactors needed for successful implementation and use of EHRs include financial support, technical support (i.e., regional extension center services), and refinement of standards.

Comparative Effectiveness Research

Carolyn M. Clancy described comparative effectiveness research as a powerful tool in providing the information needed to drive improvements in clinical care by providing information that could be used on the frontlines of treatment, and helping to make decisions more consistent, transparent, and rational. She outlined additional goals of ensuring that effectiveness data are more widely used, and promoting an open and collaborative approach to comparative effectiveness.

Capturing Clinical Data to Generate New Knowledge

Peter K. Smith suggested that clinical data be considered a knowledge utility, thus improving the ability to utilize the medical record in clinical decision making and in handoffs, improving the quality of the data, and providing essential information to better evaluate and treat the patient. He offered the example of case improvements in thoracic surgery, facilitated by a registry program for all patients introduced through the Society of Thoracic Surgeons. In order to accomplish broader use of all clinical data for new insights, he recommended a comprehensive restructuring of our clinical data collection process, including the development of universal problem lists which could facilitate patient care, quality improvement initiatives, and clinical research.

Care Culture and System Redesign

While the presentations in this session were diverse, all the strategies discussed share the central idea of shifting the current culture to one of patient-centered care through such levers as streamlined and harmonized health insurance regulation, quality and consistency in treatment with a focus on the medically complex, sharable clinical records, and medical liability reform (Chapter 9).

Team Care and Improving the Match of Clinician to Care Element

Michelle J. Lyn described strategies for using expanded teams of providers, selected to respond to local needs and resources in targeted sites across a community, to provide care earlier, more effectively, and at lower cost. Using Community Care of North Carolina (CCNC) as an example of such a strategy, she elaborated that CCNC was comprised of networks of physicians, hospitals, health departments, and social services agencies. These networks formed community-based delivery systems and collaboratively deployed teams of social workers, nurses, health educators, dieticians, community health workers, and others who work in concert with physicians to provide care management and disease management and assure appropriate access to services. Analyses estimated overall annual state savings of up to $170 million. She concluded that, despite limited experience transitioning to systems of care for an increasingly diverse, aging population, community-engaged system redesign must be part of healthcare reform.

Care Site Efficiency and Productivity Initiatives and Incentives

Drawing on the experience of the Virginia Mason Medical Center (VMMC), which applies principles from the Toyota Production System, Kim R. Pittenger explained how re-engineering of clinical services could eliminate waste and mistakes in care and thus be free of their human and dollar costs. Extrapolating nationally from VMMC's results, he estimated the sum of the clinical and patient-safety savings on a national scale from the application of such efficiency and productivity initiatives to be over $44 billion, and the operational savings through reductions in cost per relative value unit, as well as lower capital and liability costs, to be over $7 billion for medical provider groups. Similarly, Sandeep Green Vaswani described the prospects for efficiencies in reducing variability in patient flow and clinical processes. He particularly highlighted the artificial portion of variability, resulting from inappropriate management, as having negative consequences for patients, providers, private employers, and the government. Recommending what he called Variability Methodology and Operations Management, Vaswani outlined several assumptions made in calculating the potential benefits of nationwide implementation, which he estimated could range from $35 to $112 billion.

Care Site Integration Initiatives

Timothy G. Ferris discussed a 3-year Centers for Medicare & Medicaid Services care coordination demonstration based at Massachusetts General Hospital (MGH) for Medicare beneficiaries with a large number of chronic conditions. Relative to a matched control group, patients in the intervention group had lower costs, fewer admissions, lower mortality, and greater use of hospice. After 2 years, the intervention showed net savings for the enrolled population of between 4 percent and 5 percent of all healthcare costs, which translated into a 1 percent to 2 percent overall savings for the total population of Medicare beneficiaries from which the intervention patients were selected. While acknowledging that several of MGH's characteristics—integration of hospital and physician services, existing electronic medical records system, extensive primary care service network—may limit generalizability, he estimated that a similar national initiative could yield between $600 million and $1 billion in Medicare savings per year. He concluded that the apparent success of the MGH Care Management Program suggests that prospective payment for the enhanced management of high-risk patients holds some promise for reducing costs.

Information Technology Initiatives to Improve Efficiency

Focusing on interoperability and health information exchange (HIE), Ashish Jha presented background data on HIE, explaining how it could help streamline, as noted earlier, the more than 30 billion healthcare transactions occurring each year in our expensive, fragmented delivery system. Describing the main mechanism for HIE in the United States, he explained that Regional Health Information Organizations bring together independent entities in a defined geographic region to create networks that will set up an electronic health information infrastructure. However, they have struggled with issues of funding and sustainability. He also reviewed literature suggesting that widespread HIE might save nearly $80 billion in annual healthcare costs, and also explored the limitations of the methods utilized to reach the estimates. Jha cited the formation of a national strategy and standardized infrastructure protocols as keys to driving the success of HIE.

Service Capacity Restrictions

Frank A. Sloan noted that since the hospital sector is the largest single care provider, previous public policies aimed at reducing service capacity have targeted hospitals largely for this reason. Whether or not service capacity restrictions could reduce spending on hospital care in particular or on personal health services in general depended on how the healthcare system was structured, he suggested. He also discussed how, if prices were set by governments, then it may be desirable to implement policies that limit capacity, and if capacity reduction lowered such cost, then lower prices of services could be achieved. However, in the past, certificate of need programs have generally neither effectively limited capacity nor contained hospital cost growth, and their effects on patient access and quality are mixed.

Antitrust Regulations

Roger Feldman framed antitrust policy as an important tool for preserving competition, thus ensuring that markets provided goods and services at the lowest price to consumers of health care. Reviewing basic antitrust tools, he described how antitrust policy was ineffective in blocking hospital mergers because of: overly expansive definitions of the geographic and product markets for hospital care; questionable legal reasoning; and promises that the merger partners would make community payments. Suggestions to improve the impact of antitrust policy in enhancing the competitive environment included: lowering the Hart-Scott-Rodino financial triggers for pre-merger review by the Department of Justice and the Federal Trade Commission; achieving better coordination between federal and state antitrust agencies; challenging physician mergers; insisting on divestiture as a remedy; and not accepting the community payment justification for mergers.

Medical Liability Reform

Randall R. Bovbjerg suggested that conventional reforms of medical liability could be expected to reduce health spending and health insurance premiums in three ways: (1) it may directly lower malpractice premiums and other costs incurred by medical providers in responding to lawsuits; (2) it may indirectly reduce the costs of "defensive medicine," activities undertaken more for legal defense than for patient benefit; and (3) it may accrue savings from the synergy of combining tort reform with other cost-containment initiatives, both in legislation and in implementation. Based on his review of the published econometric literature, the estimated savings on premiums and defensive medicine would be approximately 0.9 percent for all personal health spending, or almost $20 billion saved in 2010 and almost $260 billion over a full decade, spread across public-sector and private-sector spending. The third type of savings, from the mutual reinforcement of malpractice reform and such other initiatives as evidence-based medicine, could well achieve synergistic savings that go further.

Transparency of Costs and Results

In this series of discussions, the presenters addressed the potential of transparency on a variety of facets of the delivery system—including cost, quality, and outcomes—to illuminate vital information for consumers, providers, and payers and stimulate savings and quality improvements (Chapter 10).

Transparency in Prices

John Santa described functional markets as relying on transparency related to comparisons, cost, and information equity to create competition. He discussed how trust in major health industry sectors has declined significantly in part because of a lack of transparency. With specific attention to transparency approaches related to benefit design, pharmaceutical purchasing, and prescribing, he said that insisting on transparency at every step in the healthcare process can contribute to a more balanced and fair market, and, when used consistently, can reduce costs and improve outcomes.

Transparency in Comparative Value of Treatment Options

Focusing on methods of reducing healthcare spending in the United States without compromising quality of care or population health, G. Scott Gazelle discussed the requirement of careful allocation of healthcare dollars and the ability of cost-effectiveness analysis (CEA) to guide those allocation decisions. CEA, where technologies, procedures, and other healthcare interventions are compared to relevant alternatives in a manner that takes into account effects on both health outcomes and costs, provides information on the relative value of competing options to patients, providers, payers, and policy makers. Citing the example of cost-effectiveness studies of human papillomavirus (HPV) testing as a primary cervical cancer screening test in combination with cervical cytology, he described how these analyses informed national and international guideline recommendations. Incorporating the CEA results, these recommendations now suggest that screening at 2- or 3-year intervals with either liquid-based cytology or combined HPV DNA testing and cytology would provide increased protection against cervical cancer while at the same time reducing the average lifetime costs associated with screening. Gazelle suggested CEA as an essential element of any comprehensive approach that seeks to maximize the benefits from our healthcare dollars.

Transparency in Comparative Value of Clinicians

Paul B. Ginsburg discussed how transparency for price and quality of services of providers has the potential to further efficiency and improve quality of care. However, he suggested that the near-term potential of these steps have been oversold. He described patient use of quality data as stymied by the dual lack of awareness of quality variation among providers and the complexity of combining numerous process measures of quality into an overall score. Continuing, he spoke of how a large impact of price transparency was dependent on provider payment reform and the insurance benefit structures that provided incentives for patients to choose more efficient providers.

Transparency in Comparative Value of Hospitals and Integrated Systems

Peter K. Lindenauer asserted that greater transparency of hospital quality and price information might improve the value of hospital care by catalyzing hospital improvement efforts, price competition, or patients' choice of better institutions. However, he indicated also that evidence is currently limited on the potential of transparency to lower costs. He suggested public reporting of readmission, complication, and healthcare-associated infection rates as offering the best hope of simultaneously lowering costs while improving the outcomes of care. Extrapolating from the benefits of the New York State Cardiac Surgery Reporting System, he presented estimates that this strategy could result in as much as $5 billion in annual savings, and might be strengthened by linking hospital payments directly to performance. He additionally suggested that while there is limited evidence for the benefits of transparency on hospital outcomes, assigning savings to transparency could be inherently problematic at some level, since reporting initiatives provide the stimulus for changes in care, but do not directly change care itself.

Transparency in Comparative Value of Insurance Companies

Margaret E. O'Kane posited that while quality transparency has stimulated gains in the quality of care delivered, significant gaps in reporting and accountability remain. She cited the percentage of patients in accountable health plans that receive a beta blocker after a heart attack as rising from 63 percent in 1996 to 98 percent in 2006. However, these improvements have been limited to the part of the industry that has either voluntarily focused on quality or been pushed into accountability. Identifying a number of reasons for this partial success, she suggested that, as healthcare costs have ballooned out of control, purchasers have increasingly selected plans based on cost of premiums or best provider discounts; many private purchasers have not rewarded high performing plans; consumers often have few or no choice of health plans; and many health plans have been ambivalent about their role in quality.

Payment and Payer-Based Strategies

Exploring the range of strategies targeting the payment and payer systems, these presentations underscored the ability of streamlined and harmonized health insurance regulation, administrative simplification and consistency, and payment redesign to focus incentives on results and value as sources of opportunities for lowering costs and improving outcomes (Chapter 11).

Paying by Anticipated Value

Harold D. Miller described widespread agreement that current methods of paying for health care contribute to both high costs and poor quality. Not only do current payment methods create strong incentives to increase the volume of services delivered, they often create barriers to delivering higher-value care and they can penalize providers for keeping people healthy, reducing errors and complications, and avoiding unnecessary services. This presentation identified alternative ways of paying for health care, from bundled payments to care warranties, which might enable and reward higher quality and lower costs. Also discussed were the types of patients, provider organizational structures, and market conditions that were most conducive to successful use of each payment approach.

Paying by Care Episode or Condition

Amita Rastogi focused on bundled payments as a tool for driving beneficial delivery system changes that could reduce costs and improve quality of health care. Citing the example of the Prometheus model, she described the development of evidence-informed case rates (ECRs) for acute events, procedures, and chronic care. ECRs are severity-adjusted, budgeted at the patient level, and encompass costs of all necessary care (physician visits, prescriptions, lab tests, imaging, etc.) over the course of an episode based on established clinical guidelines. Also discussed were allowances for potentially avoidable complications (PACs) that serve as a warranty against care defects. Based on their analysis of commercial insurance claims, as PACs represented about 10 percent of the total annual costs of care for a large national employer after modeling 13 ECRs, reducing their incidence to zero could save $355 billion annually for commercially insured plan members.

Managed Competition and Accountable Care Organizations

David R. Riemer drew on evidence from the Wisconsin State Employee Health Plan to describe health insurance exchanges as a powerful mechanism for reducing healthcare costs and improving healthcare quality. This plan provides state employees a benefit package; offers the same benefit package regardless of whether enrollees select one of several HMOs or the fee-for-service Standard Plan; and gives employees a strong incentive to choose a low-cost plan. The Dane County model—which uses an exchange—has consistently yielded premiums that are substantially lower than those in other counties. He suggested that exchanges will be effective if they meet certain criteria, including having a large number of participants to command the attention of competing health insurance companies; using powerful incentives to induce insurers to lower their premiums; and improving the quality of the health care provided by the insurers' networks of doctors, clinics, and hospitals.

Structuring Insurance Prices According to Anticipated Value

Niteesh K. Choudhry explained that value-based insurance design (VBID) utilized copayments, coinsurance, deductibles, and other similar strategies to contain healthcare spending by encouraging patients to only consume medical services with benefits greater than their costs. Extrapolating from recent literature about the efficacy of VBID, he estimated if VBID were applied nationally to five common conditions, a potential savings of more than $2 billion per year might be possible. However, he cautioned that these preliminary estimates, by necessity, aggregate groups of conditions into single disease categories, such as "heart disease," do not account for patients with more than one related condition, and do not distinguish between the impact on patients of different disease severities. Lisa Carrara described the potential of applying VBID to providers. By designating high performing specialists based on measures of clinical quality and efficiency as a method of directing consumers to make healthcare decisions based on the overall value of care, rather than just price alone, she provided estimates of a 3 to 4 percent savings in a customer's annual claims in its first year. With ready access to information on costs, treatment options, and clinical quality, she suggested that patients will work together with their physicians to decide what care is best for them—a choice based on overall value.

Payer Harmonization, Coordination, and/or Consolidation

Robin J. Thomashauer discussed how payer harmonization was already reducing administrative burden by eliminating redundant paper-based processes, and improving the accuracy, consistency, and timeliness of electronic data transactions. Current Council for Affordable Quality Healthcare (CAQH) initiatives—the Committee on Operating Rules for Information Exchange (CORE) and the Universal Provider Datasource (UPD)—have produced real results that could be tracked across a wide range of stake-holders. CORE is developing and promulgating operating rules built on national standards, such as HIPAA, to facilitate administrative data exchange and promote interoperability. Based upon a recent outcomes study, industry-wide implementation of the CORE Phase I rules could save the industry an estimated $3 billion over 3 years. Citing the success of this cross-industry, public–private collaboration, Thomashauer outlined the need for continued collaboration focused on both short- and long-term goals, coupled with the appropriate federal policy support. Complementing Thomashauer's estimates, David S. Wichmann identified a savings opportunity of $332 billion in national health expenditures over the next decade from the application of technology to administrative simplification, based on the experience of UnitedHealth Group. Ranging from automated eligibility verification to elimination of paper remittances, he outlined 12 options that would provide a strong foundation from which to advance an ongoing administrative simplification agenda. To achieve these savings and improve healthcare delivery, he urged shared, consistent action across all payers—commercial and governmental—in partnership with physicians and hospitals.

Community-Based and Transitional Care

Speakers participating in this session identified the critical role prevention and population health, as well as quality and consistency in treatment with a focus on the medically complex, could play in lowering the burden of chronic illness and improving productivity and quality of life (Chapter 12).

Care Management for Medically Complex Patients

Identifying a high-risk population that suffers from fragmentation and uncoordinated care, Kenneth E. Thorpe discussed the needs of medically complicated patients, demonstrating that patients with chronic disease were estimated to account for 75 percent of overall health spending. Yet, chronically ill patients receive just 55 percent of clinically recommended services, which he suggested may explain a nontrivial portion of morbidity and mortality. Positing that community health teams could work closely with providers to optimize patient self-management, he reviewed findings from a recent study on frail elders in transitional care that suggest a ten-year investment of $25 billion in transitional care could lead to $100 billion in savings over the same period.

Palliative Care

Diane E. Meier described palliative care as an interdisciplinary team-based model anchored in treatment of pain and other symptoms; expert communication with patients and families about the realities of the illness and achievable goals for care; and skilled coordination of care across the many settings traversed by these patients. As such, she explained that palliative care was highly adapted to serving the 23 percent of Medicare beneficiaries with five or more chronic conditions who drive over two-thirds of all Medicare spending. After describing the benefits of palliative care in terms of the major domains of quality, including patient-centeredness, benefit, safety, and efficiency, she suggested that savings associated with palliative care, once scaled to meet ongoing needs, were estimated to be nearly $5 billion per year.

Wellness and Community-Based Programs

Drawing on work of Trust for America's Health and the Urban Institute, Jeffrey Levi discussed the healthcare cost impact of community-based prevention programs that targeted some of the more expensive chronic diseases. Published literature suggested that community-based programs could lead to improvements in physical activity and nutrition, and could prevent smoking and other tobacco use. With the cost of many effective community-based programs at under $10 per person per year, Levi suggested that an investment of $10 per person per year in proven community-based prevention programs could result in a net annual savings of $2.8 billion in 1 to 2 years; $16.5 billion in 5 years; and $18.4 billion in 10 to 20 years. The 5-year savings would be accrued across payers, with $5.2 billion for Medicare, $1.9 billion for Medicaid, and $9.3 billion for private payers and out-of-pocket costs. Levi acknowledged that these estimates do not reflect the costs of implementation. He additionally noted a paradigm shift in the commitment to prevention efforts, reflected by the ARRA of 2009 investment of $650 million to introduce community-based prevention programs and study their impacts.

Entrepreneurial Strategies

In this session, the presenters considered entrepreneurial strategies and innovations, offering yet another host of pathways for increasing efficiency, enhancing quality, and containing costs (Chapter 13).

Reducing Stratified Clinician Restrictions

Jason Hwang relayed that, in the early stages of most industries, market demand for improved performance and efficiency leads to a centralization of expertise and resources. However, this centralization creates a model that constantly seeks to augment functionality at additional cost over time. In contrast, he described disruptive innovation as a process by which these centralized models are transformed into affordable and conveniently accessible resources. Examples of disruptive innovations in health care that he discussed included retail clinics and their use of nurse practitioners, online patient networks that depended on the collective wisdom of consumers, and expert systems software that enabled generalists to begin doing the work of specialists.

Retail Clinics

N. Marcus Thygeson explained that retail clinics (RCs) were designed to deliver a limited set of simple clinical services in a convenient setting and were typically staffed by mid-level providers with remote medical director oversight. With an average cost per episode in a RC of $55 less than in physician offices or urgent care, if all of the five most common RC-eligible episode types (approximately 250 episodes per 10,000 member months) were treated in RCs, commercially-insured population healthcare costs might decrease by $1.40 per member per month (PMPM), or 0.5 percent of total PMPM. Extrapolating nationally, he suggested that this represented potential savings of nearly $8 billion annually if all RC-eligible episodes were treated in retail clinics. However, he stressed that the actual savings may be lower if established providers maintain their revenue by increasing the number of visits per episode for their remaining patients, or charge more for non-retail clinic-eligible services.

Technological Innovation

Adam Darkins discussed the potential for technologies that incorporate health informatics, telehealth, and disease management to impact the outcomes and costs management of patients with chronic disease. Focusing on telehealth, he reviewed accumulating data that suggested such care coordination with home telehealth approaches could significantly reduce healthcare costs and improve access to care in rural communities. If taken to the national level and assuming the same level of savings could be achieved in non-VA health systems, implementation of telehealth applications in targeted areas for patients with chronic illness could translate to net cost savings of approximately $2 billion for Medicaid. Darkins also identified the associated re-engineering of the underlying care delivery process as critical to the adoption of this technology.

Lessons from Abroad

In considering international efforts to improve quality while lowering costs, this presentation focused on the need for payment redesign to focus incentives on results and value, medical liability reform, and patient-centered care (Chapter 7).

International Examples

Drawing on examples from other countries, Gerard F. Anderson suggested that payment reforms, no fault malpractice insurance, and care coordination are transplantable strategies for lowering costs and improving outcomes in this country. Noting that specialists in the United States earn up to 300 percent more than those in other countries, that prices for branded drugs cost up to twice as much, and that hospital stays are up to 200 percent more expensive, he suggested that cost control mechanisms in other nations such as Germany have helped control spending growth and could yield significant savings if applied here. With respect to differences in medical liability costs, Anderson said that while Canada and the United Kingdom have similar types of malpractice insurance as the United States and similar rates of litigation and award levels, the no fault malpractice model in New Zealand has resulted in lower premiums and fewer lawsuits. Finally, he also discussed Germany's focus on care coordination for individuals with chronic conditions and their provider, payer and consumer incentives, which together have lead to decreasing rates of hospitalizations for this population.

WORKSHOP THREE: THE POLICY AGENDA

The third workshop, The Policy Agenda, considered the following six policies to lower costs and improve outcomes:

- Payments for value over volume;
- Care for medically complex patients;
- Delivery system integration;
- Improved delivery system efficiency;
- Administrative simplification; and
- Consumer-focused strategies.

In her workshop keynote, Karen Davis discussed priorities for policy options to achieve cost control and affordable coverage for all. She identified the goals of health reform as: slowing growth in health spending; creating incentives for providers to take broader accountability for patient care, outcomes, and resource use; providing rewards for improved care coordination among providers; and putting in place an infrastructure to support providers in improving quality and efficiency. She discussed how these goals are driven by the current state of affairs, in which 21 percent of adults report going to the emergency room within the past 2 years for a condition that could have been treated in the office, as well as the existing three-fold spread between those in the lowest ($947) and highest quartiles ($2,911) for risk-adjusted spending for hospital readmissions after coronary bypass surgeries.

Referencing the recommendations of the Commonwealth Fund's report titled *A High Performance Health System for the United States: An Ambitious Agenda for the Next President* (The Commonwealth Fund Commission on a High Performance Health System, 2007), Davis focused particular attention on the importance of aligning financial incentives to enhance value. In discussing fundamental payment reform that rewarded physicians and other providers for achieving quality, she cited examples of successful experiments such as those at Geisinger Health System. Based on their report, the Commonwealth Fund estimated that significant savings could be achieved from implementation of their policy recommendations, with a potential of $123 billion over a decade from instituting bundled payment policies, $83 billion over 10 years from strengthening primary care and care coordination, and $70 billion from promoting HIT.

Following Davis' keynote address, the meeting turned to an update and discussion of the estimates from the previous two workshops (see "Pulling the Numbers Together" below), followed by a presentation by Joseph R. Antos on the analytical framework used by CBO in developing estimates of the impact of potential legislation on the federal budget. Known as the "score" of a proposed bill, the CBO cost estimate explains how the proposal affects federal outlays and revenues over a 5 or 10 year horizon. Depending on the specifics of the proposal, he explained that CBO may use data from Medicare, Medicaid, and other federal programs; survey data (including surveys of individuals, such as the Medicare Current Beneficiary Survey and the Medical Expenditure Panel Survey, and surveys of providers and insurers); information from clinical and delivery system experiments; and other sources of data on the health system, demographics, and the economy. Utilizing a variety of information sources, CBO analysts develop their modeling assumptions based on peer-reviewed literature; unpublished studies from reputable sources; direct observation of trends in the health-care market; comparisons with previous analyses by CBO and others of similar proposals; and consultation with experts, including staff from the

Centers for Medicare & Medicaid Services (CMS), insurance actuaries, medical leaders, academics, and others.

Subsequent presenters turned to discussions of policy options, issues of implementation timing and phasing, the critical co-factors for success, and the options to minimize political barriers. Brief summaries of the individual presentations are presented below.

Payments for Value over Volume

While focusing specifically on bundled payments for providers, the presenters in this session revealed that although some practices are promising, there remain significant challenges for implementation (Chapter 15).

Options for Payment Redesign to Focus on Episode, Condition, or Capitation

John M. Bertko focused on the experience of the private sector with bundled payments, reviewing experiments that have occurred over the past two decades. After describing the successes of Geisinger Health System's ProvenCare™ program, under which hospital and physicians are paid a global fee, and insurers' bundled transplant programs in centers of excellence, he contrasted this with a discussion of failures, including what was called (in the late 1990s) "contact capitation" and a somewhat similar approach by the start-up firm HealthMarket. While bundled payments for acute episodes offered promise of incentives for efficiency, he suggested that there are still many unresolved questions about the scale of this promise and the practical mechanics of provider arrangements.

Complementing this presentation, Linda M. Magno discussed the experience of CMS with bundled payments. She cited the example of Medicare's inpatient prospective payment system (IPPS) for hospitals, which represented a significant step in the direction of paying a uniform price for similar services regardless of where such services were rendered and incented hospitals to improve efficiency. IPPS resulted in reduced lengths of stay and, for at least some period of time, limited investment in new technologies to those expected to be cost-reducing or revenue-enhancing. However, much of the reduction in length of stay was accompanied by a steady rise in the supply and utilization of post-acute services, for which Medicare makes additional payments over and above the diagnosis-related group price. She also drew on Medicare's experiences with three bundled payment demonstrations, indicating lessons learned and their implications for future bundled payment endeavors.

Issues for Clinicians

George J. Isham highlighted four projects in Minnesota related to bundled care as a means of demonstrating provider engagement issues. From these initiatives, he offered several lessons learned, explaining that designing and implementing bundled payment was complex and resource intensive, and that payment reform that moved in the direction of bundled payment had to be intimately associated with delivery system reform. He suggested that gaining the right balance between the roles of legislators, expert input, and engagement of physicians in local pilots may be important to successful national implementation. He additionally emphasized that the design of bundled payment models requires clear objectives from policy makers, input from providers and others, and technical assistance on management and quality improvement at the local level.

Issues for Patients

Nancy Davenport-Ennis indicated that bundled payment systems are aligned conceptually with patient interests in improved outcomes and lower healthcare costs. However, she cautioned that the selection of which services and conditions would benefit most from bundling required careful consideration. For broad disease areas like cancer, which do not have clear boundaries between beginning, intervention, and end, she suggested that bundling would need to include robust tiers of weighted payments and outliers in order to ensure patient access to care was not compromised. In considering how patients could be involved in bundled payment systems, she cited Geisinger Health System's inclusion of a "patient compact" that was designed to engage patients in ensuring favorable outcomes. In addition to ensuring recognition of variability of disease through the use of weighted payments based on factors such as age, weight, ethnicity, and co-morbidities, she suggested that successful bundling systems must also find the proper balance between saving money and improving patient outcomes and care while continuing to allow for evolving personalization of health care.

Care for Medically Complex Patients

To explore the solutions needed to face these mounting challenges, presenters in this session discussed policy initiatives to facilitate care of the growing population of medically complex patients, emphasizing patient-centeredness, payment redesign, quality and consistency in treatment with a focus on the medically complex, and prevention at personal and population levels (Chapter 16).

Approaches That Work

Arnold Milstein explained that methods to lower per capita healthcare spending and improve clinical outcomes for medically complex patients have been demonstrated. However, many efforts to use provider payments to achieve these two aims in care for medically complex patients have failed. He identified two keys to success in payer efforts to date. The first involved incentives to primary care teams to intensify within- and between-visit care for patients at highest risk of near-term ER visits and unplanned inpatient admissions. A second offered incentives to hospitals to standardize inpatient care via checklists, care bundles, more systematic applications of process engineering tools, and/or assuring at least 8 hours of daily onsite (or telemediated) monitoring of ICU patients by intensivists.

Special Case of Palliative Care

Given considerable data suggesting that care for patients living with serious illness, and their families, is in need of improvement, R. Sean Morrison discussed palliative care as a method of providing the interdisciplinary care coordination and team-driven continuity of care needed to respond to the episodic and long-term nature of chronic, multifaceted illnesses. However, the number of palliative care programs in U.S. hospitals with over 50 beds was just over 50 percent in 2008. In order for palliative care to be accessible to all patients with serious illness and their families, he urged consideration of a number of key initiatives: education of patients, families, and healthcare professionals of the benefits of palliative care; emphasis that palliative care is not synonymous with end-of-life care; additional resources for workforce development to train sufficient numbers of specialists to effectively provide palliative care to patients and families in need; patient-oriented and health services research; and reimbursement structures that promote team-based care.

Issues for Healthcare Organizations

If the twin aims of lowering costs and improving population health are to be achieved, Ronald A. Paulus suggested, value-based payment models must move beyond payment for units of work or effort, and instead reward demonstrated patient- and population-level clinical impact and outcomes. He described a new approach at Geisinger Health System that seeks to optimize the closure rate for patients' "care gaps" (i.e., specific, patient-centric clinical needs) and facilitate teamwork between medical home-based primary care physicians and specialists. When supplemented by an electronic health record with enhanced decision support, population-level data, and integrated analytics, he explained that this approach can produce marked progress in patient and population outcomes. It could also serve as a point of reference for those seeking to develop value-based payment models structured to encourage innovation, enhance patient experience, improve clinical quality, and contain costs.

Policy Needs

Anand K. Parekh identified several policy areas that could further support tertiary prevention in individuals with multiple concurrent chronic conditions. As medically complex patients have often been excluded from participation in randomized controlled clinical trials, he suggested that the external validity and generalizability of these studies to this population are limited. While identifying the importance of health professions training in the care of medically complex patients, he explained that many current evidence-based guidelines focus on individual chronic diseases, thus disregarding the coexistence of other chronic conditions in patients, and putting patients at risk of drug-drug or drug-disease adverse interactions. He additionally discussed patient engagement as playing a central role in patient management of their own care and provider payment reform as essential to the success of incentives for care coordination and management.

Delivery System Integration

Highlighting the benefits of streamlined and harmonized health insurance regulation, payment redesign, and secure, sharable clinical records, the presentations in this session targeted delivery system integration and connectivity as methods of lowering costs and improving outcomes (Chapter 17).

Organizational Initiatives to Reduce Fragmentation

John Toussaint defined care fragmentation as the lack of the necessary resources available to the patient to manage his or her condition in a timely fashion. He explained that the current care delivery system is not designed for consumers but rather for providers and hospitals, and contended that this was the result of a lack of fundamental understanding of what constitutes value from the patient perspective. Elaborating on current initiatives to improve care coordination, he cited multiple examples of success. Group Health of Puget Sound reduced emergency room visits by 29 percent by redesigning their clinical services. Thedacare's Collaborative

Care Unit lowered inpatient care costs by 25 percent. Gunderson Lutheran's care coordination process included a focus on end-of-life care, resulting in costs per Medicare enrollee that were 50 percent less expensive than the national average.

Payment Incentives to Promote Integration

Drawing on the work of the Medicare Payment Advisory Commission, Mark E. Miller described Medicare's fee-for-service (FFS) payment system as one that rewards more care, without regard to the value of that care. In addition, Medicare's payment system creates separate payment "silos" (e.g., inpatient hospitals, physicians, post-acute care providers) and fails to encourage coordination among providers within a silo or across silos. When discussing evidence demonstrating that care coordination can improve quality, he suggested that Medicare must develop new payment methods that will reward efficient use of limited resources and encourage the effective integration of care. This presentation specifically focused on approaches to payment that would encourage greater coordination of care, resulting in higher quality and lower Medicare spending: reducing preventable hospital readmissions, increasing the use of bundled payments, and holding accountable care organizations responsible for the cost and quality of the care their patients receive.

Building on these ideas, Harold S. Luft outlined alternatives to the current system that could facilitate coordination of inpatient and similar interventional care as well as coordination and effective management of ongoing chronic care. Focusing on proposals for medical homes, bundling, and evidence-based practice, he explained that these initiatives align incentives for value-enhancing care and facilitate the development and spread of the information needed by clinicians to deliver that care. Unlike global capitation, however, they retain aspects of fee-for-service where that payment approach is not problematic, thus reducing opposition from those resistant to change, avoiding the productivity problems faced in large organizations, allowing their application in communities in which highly integrated systems may be either infeasible or an antitrust concern, and engendering flexibility as medical technology and knowledge changes.

"Virtual Integration" and the Promise of Health Information Technology

Andrew M. Wiesenthal explored the potential for increased use of EHRs, coupled with effective, standards-based HIE, surmising that together they could counteract the powerful forces contributing to poor integration. Promoting EHR deployment and meaningful use are appropriate first steps for the country to take, he elaborated, followed closely by targeting improved outcomes in chronic diseases. He estimated that improving system integration at an appropriate regional level will likely require 5 to 10 years once the work has started. National integration would be much more difficult, lengthier, and largely unneeded by most patients. He identified the business and public health communities as crucial participants for this effort. At the same time, if integration is to be achieved, he asserted that regulatory and competitive barriers, along with patient fears of data misuse, must be addressed.

Improved Delivery System Efficiency

From using market forces to effect change by empowering consumers to make informed choices to redefining who provides health care, the presenters in this session discussed innovations to improve delivery system efficiency (Chapter 18).

Policies That Promote Clinician Efficiencies

Mary D. Naylor asserted that enhancing the effectiveness and efficiency of the U.S. healthcare system was dependent upon maximizing the contributions of healthcare professionals who are not physicians. She identified a number of current barriers which limit appropriate use of such providers, including federal and state laws and regulations; opposition from healthcare systems, professional medical groups, and managed care organizations; reimbursement and other payment policies; and exclusion from demonstrations proposed as part of health reform. Policies options outlined by Naylor included: advancing regulatory reform that would revise state "scope of practice" laws where unnecessarily restrictive; including qualified providers in testing of proposed system redesign and payment reform demonstrations; payment reform that emphasizes the team as the payment unit and reinforces the team's accountability for individual and population health while promoting fair compensation for licensed independent practitioners by all payers; implementation and enforcement of "any willing provider" laws in all states; and promotion of research assessing the value and comparative effectiveness of innovative care and payment with a variety of providers.

Policies That Promote System Efficiencies

Steven J. Spear suggested that large opportunities currently exist to advance quality, access, and cost simultaneously by focusing on care delivery. Despite significant disparities between the quality of providers, patients and payers cannot distinguish which providers provide the highest quality care at affordable cost. Focusing on empowering patients and payers with this information, he explained that transparency has the ability to promote efficiency within the healthcare system.

Administrative Simplification

The presenters in this session discussed promising policy solutions to facilitate administrative simplification, ranging from leveraging technology to standardizing reporting requirements (Chapter 19).

Accelerating Administrative Streamlining Among Payers

Lewis G. Sandy reviewed the significant $332 billion opportunity in administrative savings identified by UnitedHealth Group, along with additional estimates from the peer-reviewed literature. To realize these opportunities, he suggested the following policy actions: policies that promote "spread" of existing standards and capabilities; policies that promote electronic connectivity and transaction automation; and polices that support multipayer capability development. He emphasized the importance of interoperability and progressive maturation of system capability, as opposed to emphasizing standardization alone, and the role of public–private sector coordination and harmonization in accelerating these advancements.

Accelerating Administrative Streamlining Among Providers

Linda L. Kloss stated that past efforts at healthcare administrative simplification have often not only failed to reduce costs, but have actually added complexity and cost. Real improvements and cost reductions require an end-to-end view of the business processes, not only within, but across, sectors and entities, and a commitment to uniform and standard process and continuous improvement. Drawing on the work of the Healthcare Administrative Simplification Coalition, she focused on four processes with the potential to reduce costs for providers and payers and improve service to purchasers and consumers: (1) practitioner credentialing, (2) insurance eligibility, (3) standard insurance identification cards, and (4) prior authorization. She also identified policy governance, uniform standards, education on process and conformance, and continuous improvement as four common elements among recommendations relating to claims and payment, quality reporting, terminologies and classifications, and other critical healthcare business processes.

Policy Opportunities to Accelerate Administrative Streamlining Initiatives

Harry Reynolds suggested that, through the tracking and the reporting of actual operational changes, industry-driven efforts to bring lasting change to the administrative aspects of health care were demonstrating their ability to reduce costs and increase efficiencies. On the other hand, he also suggested that, although many in the industry are working to gain greater industry adoption of these efforts, significant challenges exist with regard to how to integrate these efforts across the healthcare system to achieve all-payer administrative simplification, public and private alike. Discussing the specific challenges and potential opportunities demonstrated through two initiatives—the Universal Provider Datasource and the Committee on Operating Rules for Information Exchange—he emphasized the critical nature of ensuring these efforts continue to be aligned with federal HIT policies, the necessity of multistakeholder support, and the barriers posed by the inevitable changes to current business practices.

Consumer-Directed Policies

To further explore the variety of policies and perspectives central to effectively engaging consumers in choosing higher-value services, panelists in this session explored such policy tools as value-based purchasing and transparency (Chapter 20).

Issues and Opportunities for Consumers

Jennifer Sweeney reviewed research revealing that consumers are seeking partnerships with their healthcare providers, information and guidance about conditions and treatments, tools and support to care for themselves, and open communication that encourages questions, dialogue, and treatment preferences and respects cultural differences. She suggested that meeting consumers' needs and recognizing their places on the activation continuum must drive any engagement strategy. However, she proposed that the healthcare system has not yet provided the tools or incentives to enable patients to fully engage in their care. Stakeholders must recognize that the majority of consumers are unaware of quality deficiencies in our healthcare system and are insulated from healthcare costs. As tools to create delivery system changes that address the needs and desires of consumers, she highlighted options including implementation of patient-centered care models, use of patient experience surveys, changes in benefit design, and consumer-friendly performance reporting.

Issues and Opportunities for Insurers

With the theoretical impact of moving all care to providers in the top tier of efficiency and quality ranging up to 5 percent of total medical costs, Dick Salmon suggested that achieving these theoretical potentials required providing patients with credible information that is easy to obtain and integrated into the healthcare experience. Additionally, individuals must have reasonable access to preferred providers and benefit incentives. He stressed that barriers to progress include assisting the transition from the customary method of selecting a healthcare professional based on reputation to a model based, in part, on comparison of reliable information on quality and cost. Enabling and rewarding individuals to choose the existing highest value provider of care offered an immediate impact on the quality and affordability of health care for individuals today, and stimulated all healthcare providers to improve in the future. As the stimulus for future improvement based on consumer choice was limited by access issues and provider loyalty, he asserted that payment reform remains essential.

Issues and Opportunities for Purchasers

Building on these concepts, Dolores L. Mitchell described the increasing pressures faced by purchasers to engage their employees in the business of wellness and prudent healthcare choices. By demonstrating how one public employer attempted to engage both employees and providers by analyzing provider performance and giving employees financial incentives to use the results (ranging from premium increases to high deductible plans), she suggested that transparency without consequences was necessary but not sufficient to affect the delivery system. She stated that the road to meaningful patient engagement was steep but should be engaged with particular attention to shared sacrifice in the short term and shared responsibility in the long term.

A Look Back at the Numbers

J. Michael McGinnis, in comments in the "look back" session summarizing the issues and estimates from the first two meetings and in the wrap-up concluding session of the third meeting offered a broad preliminary overview of what might be observed by simply examining totals for the estimates presented in the various workshop presentations and in the background literature review prepared to inform the discussions. After cautioning that the authors' estimates were themselves still works in progress—with many gaps, overlaps, and areas of uncertainty—he noted that taking, as a constrained first approximation, the *lower bounds* of the estimates from the source material allowed some interesting observations.

First, at the very highest level—aggregate excess costs systemwide—he noted that estimates made from four analytically distinct approaches came to roughly similar approximations for the nation's total excess healthcare costs. Specifically, looking at regional variations in care costs, the Dartmouth group estimated overall excess expenditures to be about 30 percent of national health expenditures (Wennberg et al., 2002), translating to approximately $750 billion in 2009; the analysis by McKinsey Global Institute (Farrell et al., 2008) would indicate that the excess U.S. expenditure relative to OECD countries to be approximately $760 billion (adjusted to 2009 total expenditure levels); the lower bound totals of estimates of excess expenditures identified from workshop discussions would amount to about $765 billion in 2009; and the estimated possible savings (lower bound, corrected for obvious overlaps) from full implementation of effective strategies would in 2009 be in the range of $550 billion. He also emphasized that such estimates are virtually all unvalidated extrapolations, based on assumptions from limited observations.

McGinnis noted that while many of the workshop calculations were similar to those published elsewhere and summarized in the background materials developed for the series, others were quite different, both from each other and from other published material, with respect to variations in methodology and scope of analyses—e.g., federal savings locus compared to societal locus; focus on public and/or private insurance beneficiaries; and annual versus multiyear timeframes. For example, Owens estimated that a program designed to reduce the incidence of uncoordinated care could result in $271 billion in annual national savings by 2013, while Berenson and colleagues, who looked only at dually-eligible Medicare and Medicaid beneficiaries, developed a 10-year estimate of $200 billion savings from a national effort to improve care coordination (Berenson et al., 2009). He also noted the ongoing field debate about how to best assess the returns from investments in preventive services and community-oriented chronic disease management (CBO, 2004; The Commonwealth Fund, 2009; DeVol et al., 2007; Elmendorf, 2009a; Russell, 2009; UnitedHealth Group, 2009), with many emphasizing that shortfalls in identified dollar savings does not signify that prevention lacks either cost-effectiveness or value.

Taking these various issues, differences, and analytic fragilities into account, McGinnis used the "lower bound of estimates" approach to summarize in broad terms the aggregate excess expenditures discussed at the workshop, both by the six categories that make up the broad domains of excess and by the component elements discussed for each of the domains, noting that within domain estimates often focused on only one aspect of the component elements. Approximations using this approach sum to 2009 totals of about $210 billion in excess health costs from unnecessary services, $130 billion from inefficiently delivered services, $190 billion from excess administrative costs, $105 billion from prices that are too high, $55 billion from missed prevention opportunities, and $75 billion from fraud (Box S-2).

With respect to the possibility of reducing excess expenditures by broader application of strategies showing early promise in limited studies, McGinnis underscored the difference between the level of unnecessary ex-

BOX S-2
Excess Cost Domain Estimates:
Lower bound totals from workshop discussions*

UNNECESSARY SERVICES   **Total excess = $210 B***
- Overuse: services beyond evidence-established levels
- Discretionary use beyond benchmarks
  - Defensive medicine
- Unnecessary choice of higher cost services

INEFFICIENTLY DELIVERED SERVICES   **Total excess = $130 B***
- Mistakes—medical errors, preventable complications
- Care fragmentation
- Unnecessary use of higher cost providers
- Operational inefficiencies at care delivery sites
  - Physician offices
  - Hospitals

EXCESS ADMINISTRATIVE COSTS   **Total excess = $190 B***
- Insurance-related administrative costs beyond benchmarks
  - Insurers
  - Physician offices
  - Hospitals
  - Other providers
- Insurer administrative inefficiencies
- Care documentation requirement inefficiencies

PRICES THAT ARE TOO HIGH   **Total excess = $105 B***
- Service prices beyond competitive benchmarks
  - Physician services
    i. Specialists
    ii. Generalists
  - Hospital services
- Product prices beyond competitive benchmarks
  - Pharmaceuticals
  - Medical devices
  - Durable medical equipment

MISSED PREVENTION OPPORTUNITIES   **Total excess = $55 B***
- Primary prevention
- Secondary prevention
- Tertiary prevention

FRAUD   **Total excess = $75 B***
- All sources—payer, clinician, patient

---

*Lower bound totals of various estimates, adjusted to 2009 total expenditure level.

penditures and the ability to capture the returns. For example, it was noted that, while an independent estimate from outside the scientific literature calculated the costs of defensive medicine at $210 billion (PriceWaterhouse-Coopers, 2008), Bovbjerg's review of the econometric literature led him to suggest that tort reform would reduce national health spending by approximately 0.9 percent, or about $20 billion in 2010. Further testament to the complexity of interpreting the estimates is that Bovbjerg's estimate focused primarily on the direct impact of reform, as opposed to the indirect influence of liability dynamics on clinicians' decisions.

Similarly, he noted that several studies on potential savings highlighted by Kaushal and Jha projected significant national savings from nationwide implementation of HIT, but CBO cautioned that, while many policy makers believe that HIT will be a necessary tool in improving the efficiency and quality of health care in the United States, overoptimistic assumptions may temper the magnitude of those estimates (CBO, 2008).

In referring to several presentations that suggested the potential for considerable savings from payment reform, McGinnis noted that Rastogi's savings estimate of $355 billion for the commercially insured from implementation of bundled payments was similar to a published estimate of $301 billion in savings from utilization of bundled payments for acute care episodes (The Commonwealth Fund, 2009); but he also noted that both estimates required validation with structured studies and experiments. It was also suggested that many potential sources of savings need more consideration than was able to be given at the workshops.

Additional areas suggested for consideration both in terms of targets and strategies included the issues such as costs of fraud and abuse, which has been estimated to cost 3 to 10 percent of total health spending (FBI, 2007), as well as the implications of the current patent system on the prices of new and emerging technologies.

Opportunities to Get to 10 Percent

The conversations and presentations occurring over the course of the workshop series, including a panel discussion with economic experts Elizabeth A. McGlynn, David O. Meltzer, and Peter J. Neumann, clearly indicated that each domain was significant, the estimates were large, and that multifaceted strategies were required to lower spending adequately over the long run. Meltzer additionally suggested that, based on the presentation analytics, that unnecessary services provided the largest area of inefficiency and waste. Meanwhile, McGlynn expressed the view that, based on modeling for Massachusetts, payment reform was the most likely to have significant impact on lowering costs, as compared to infrastructure improvements and delivery system interventions (Box S-3).

BOX S-3
Estimated 10-Year Health Cost Savings, 2010-2020
Selected approaches: one analyst's model

	Cumulative Change in National Health Spending	
	Low	High
Bundled payments	−0.1%	−5.4%
Hospital-rate regulation	0.0%	−2.0%
Health IT	+0.8%	−1.5%
Disease management	+1.0%	−1.3%
Medical homes	+0.4%	−1.2%
Retail clinics	0.0%	−0.6%
Expanded NP/PA use	−0.3%	−0.5%
Benefit design	+0.2%	−0.3%

NOTE: IT = information technology; NP = nurse practitioner; PA = physician assistant.
SOURCE: Adapted from Eibner et al., 2009. Controlling Health Care Spending in Massachusetts. Online by Eibner et al. Copyright 2009 by RAND Corporation. Reproduced with permission of RAND Corporation in the format Other book via Copyright Clearance Center.

On the other hand, panelists cautioned that estimates, extrapolated of necessity from "thought experiments," must be interpreted with caution as they may not be as informed from real life experiences and observations. While the savings benefits of infrastructure elements such as HIT and CER may be uncertain, McGlynn posited that these very tools were necessary to allow expansion of the delivery system's capacity to engage in delivery system reform. Meltzer and Neumann also suggested that incrementalism—the need for multiple small savings decisions over a single large decision—will be necessary to achieve 10 percent savings. While they indicated that the estimates needed additional refinement to account for overlaps, cross-integration, and the wave of emerging medical technologies, McGlynn also asserted that the lack of evidence supporting any particular strategy does not necessarily reflect a lack of value.

This final point was particularly relevant in the discussion of bundled payments and payment reform, as many major examples of bundling success, such as those of Geisinger and Kaiser Permanente, occur within the context of vertical integration of providers. Therefore, the discussants underscored that it remains unclear how bundled payments could be operationalized outside this formal organizational structure. Yet payment reform was thought to be so critical to delivery system reform that the panelists and many other attendees advocated expanding ongoing pilots to test its viability within non-vertical organizational structures.

The Policy Priorities and Strategies

The third workshop's concluding panel, composed of Mark B. McClellan, Joseph Onck, and Dean Rosen, specifically considered the issue of cost control in the context of current health policy discussions. McClellan spoke of the need to focus on four interrelated pillars which provide a broad framework for the discussion on costs and quality: (1) better information and tools to be more effective; (2) provider payments that reward improvements in quality and reductions in cost growth, provide support for healthcare delivery reforms that save money, and emphasize disease prevention and better coordination of care; (3) reform of health insurance markets and restructuring of government subsidies to create competition and improve incentives around value improvement rather than risk selection; and (4) greater support for individual patients for improving their health and lowering overall healthcare costs, including incentives for achieving measurable health goals. He further emphasized an idea frequently heard throughout the workshop, that reform efforts must engage a varied and differentiated approach rather than focusing on one area. Onek built on this idea, further suggesting that compartmentalizing reform facilitates blockage of reform politically. Strategically packaging reform initiatives allows a broader coalition to come in support of reform legislation. In addition to focusing on payment reform, Rosen additionally advocated further discussion on individual responsibility and personal investment as critical as consumers and providers jointly work to improve health and the untapped potential of medical liability reform to lower costs.

WORKSHOP FOUR: GETTING TO 10 PERCENT

Building on the discussions of the preceding workshops, a knowledgeable group of authorities from different stakeholder sectors convened to explore in greater detail the priority elements and strategies key to achieving 10 percent savings in healthcare expenditures within 10 years, without compromising health status, quality of care, or valued innovation. Participants, whose backgrounds drew from their experience as providers, payers, purchasers, health economists, researchers, quality analysts, and regulators, included Michael Bailit of Bailit Health Purchasing, Maureen Bisognano of the Institute for Healthcare Improvement, David M. Cutler of Harvard University, Wendy Everett of New England Healthcare Institute,

Richard J. Gilfillan of Geisinger Health System, Dolores L. Mitchell of the Massachusetts Group Insurance Commission, Meredith B. Rosenthal of Harvard University, Jonathan S. Skinner of Dartmouth College, John Toussaint of ThedaCare Center for Healthcare Value, and Reed V. Tuckson of UnitedHealth Group.

As the participants considered the opportunities present within the current delivery system to lower costs and improve outcomes, the substantial scale of the inefficiencies was underscored. While the attendees discussed published literature and earlier workshop presentations indicating that 20 to 30 percent of current expenditures could be trimmed without consequences for quality or outcomes (Fisher et al., 2003), certain attendees offered the view that, based on their experiences with ongoing improvement initiatives, the amount of waste present in the healthcare system may even be greater, perhaps in some circumstances and settings as much as 50 percent. As an example, the findings of the Health Care Value Leaders Network were discussed. Two of these findings were that: (1) 80 to 90 percent of steps in the care process were not value-additive, and (2) with the application of the Toyota Production System to streamline clinical services within an institution, systematic waste reduction could possibly trim as much as 50 percent of costs, while simultaneously improving quality.

The attendees discussed priority areas of opportunity, such as avoidable hospitalizations and readmissions and the provision of unnecessary services. They focused on high-yield strategies, ranging from decreasing the costs of episodes of care to medical liability reform to shared decision-making, as well as considering care-related costs, administrative costs, and related reforms. Several insights were offered by multiple individual attendees on the common elements of successful strategies:

- *Reorientation to patient-centered value* among all stakeholders (patients, providers, payers, manufacturers, and regulators) is necessary, and eliminating the inefficiencies and waste replete in the costs of care and healthcare administration begins with the basics: better attention to patient needs and perspectives, and payment mechanisms that drive the delivery of value over volume. However, it was also emphasized that the rewards involved must be quite large in comparison with the income at stake for providers if the effort is to both cover the implementation costs and justify the resources involved in maintaining a coordinated effort to minimize costs and improve outcomes.
- *Payment reform* provides a critical tool to realign economic incentives within the delivery system. Additionally, targeting both utilization and pricing of clinical services is needed to ensure the

full savings potential of any bundle of strategies to lower costs and improve outcomes.

- *Multimodality* should characterize health reform plans because while payment reform appears to be the most likely to yield near- to mid-term savings, infrastructure elements such as health information technology and comparative effectiveness research are necessary to facilitate and amplify the effectiveness of payment reforms. In particular, nonmedical industries provide many instructive lessons regarding successful cost-lowering practices, including use of data to inform quality improvements, incentive structures that reward value creation, and worker-driven processes and culture.

- *Specificity* with regard to policies, responsible actors, and assumptions enables focus of initiatives, not just in legislation but also through institutional leadership and public–private partnerships at both state and regional levels.

- *Incrementalism*—the need for multiple small savings decisions related to re-aligned incentives and improved system efficiency—rather than a single large decision—will be necessary to achieve 10 percent savings. Apart from large savings likely to be possible from streamlining and harmonizing administrative claims forms and reporting requirements, success of the broad reform approaches required will likely depend on smaller gains—targeting utilization, pricing, and delivery—in each of the many strategic loci.

- *Transparency and accountability* across public and private sectors can foster efficiency and quality improvement initiatives by providers, informed provider selection by patients, and value-based payments by payers.

- *Collaboration* among all those affected by healthcare reforms, including subspecialty provider societies, payers, and patients, is required to overcome inertia and fear of change.

Considering the Opportunities

Participants reviewed the range of strategies explored throughout the workshop series and, working in small groups followed by open discussion, considered opportunities for strategies aimed at providers, patients, and payers. Their discussion centered on care-related costs, administrative costs, and related reforms. Within each of these broad categories, they considered an array of specific initiatives as well as the requirements and assumptions inherent to each. In addition, the participants discussed their views on the approximate range of savings that might be achieved through implementation of these strategies, drawing on workshop presentations and their own experiences.

Payment reform was discussed throughout the meeting as a necessary and potent component of a value-driven agenda to lower costs and improve outcomes. Many of the participants observed that payment reform may be implemented in a variety of forms, ranging from bundled payments to global payments and salaries for providers, but they emphasized payment reform as a tool and an underlying requirement for achieving many of the goals discussed at the meeting. For example, to stimulate initiatives to reduce medical errors, several attendees suggested that creation of bundled payments for hospitalizations include the costs of readmissions due to any cause within 30 days. Another form of payment reform akin to pay-for-performance included linking a portion of provider payments to documented use of decision aids to encourage shared decision-making. Regardless of the form, payment reform was noted throughout the meeting by various individuals as fundamental to aligning provider incentives with quality and efficiency.

In the discussions, the participants individually identified high-yield savings opportunities based on their own experiences. The ten cost-reduction opportunities explored in greater detail during the meeting focused primarily on care-related costs, but also included administrative costs and related reforms (Box S-4).

While acknowledging that substantial additional analytic work was required to refine and strengthen the analytics, based on estimates provided throughout previous workshops on excess costs, and informed by their own individual knowledge bases, the sum total of the individual opinions of the various participants, speaking not for all in the group but to their own areas of expertise, resulted in first approximations of $360 billion to $460 billion in annual savings, which might be achieved by 2018 (in 2009 dollars). Across the areas noted in Box S-4, participants expressed personal opinions on the range of savings opportunities, including $8 billion to $12 billion from preventing medical errors, $44 billion to $48 billion from preventing avoidable hospital admissions, $16 billion to $20 billion from preventing avoidable hospital readmissions, $38 billion to $80 billion from improving hospital efficiency, $32 billion to $53 billion from decreasing the costs of care episodes, $9 billion to $20 billion from improving targeting of costly services, $6 billion to $9 billion from increasing shared decision-making, $181 billion from utilizing common billing and claims forms, $20 billion to $30 billion from medical liability reform, and $5 billion to $10 billion from preventing fraud and abuse. To account for the increased primary care practice costs necessary to achieve implementation of several of the strategies discussed, several participants suggested that a one-third offset be employed, yielding a total savings of approximately $240 billion

BOX S-4
Estimated Health Cost Savings
Selected approaches: individual perspectives

	Estimated Savings in Year 10	
	Low	High
CARE-RELATED COSTS		
• Prevent medical errors	$8 B	$12 B
• Prevent avoidable hospital admissions	$44 B	$48 B
• Prevent avoidable hospital readmissions	$16 B	$20 B
• Improve hospital efficiency	$38 B	$80 B
• Decrease costs of episodes of care	$32 B	$53 B
• Improve targeting of costly services	$9 B	$20 B
• Increase shared decision-making	$6 B	$9 B
ADMINISTRATIVE COSTS		
• Use common billing and claims forms	$181 B	
RELATED REFORMS		
• Medical liability reform	$20 B	$30 B
• Prevent fraud and abuse	$5 B	$10 B

to $310 billion annually. Additionally, participants pointed out that the estimates discussed had not accounted for implementation and overhead costs.

Additional Considerations

The rising epidemic of obesity, an aging population with an increasing burden of chronic illness, and the influence of current health behaviors on future health status were also cited as considerations during the conversations. With levels of obesity projected to exceed 40 percent by 2015 (Wang and Beydoun, 2007) and over 80 million Americans expected to have multiple co-morbidities by 2020 (Anderson and Horvath, 2002), Cutler and Tuckson underscored the importance of considering how health demographic trends would impact future healthcare expenditures and thus the priority strategies to address them. Given the connection between health behaviors and these health trends, including the rising levels of multiple co-occurring chronic illnesses and the low rate of recommended preventive care, Everett and Mitchell drew attention to the issue of prevention, including community health programs that encourage healthy eating habits in schools, anti-tobacco legislation, and primary through tertiary prevention. Acknowledging that uncertainty exists about the cost effectiveness of many prevention initiatives, Tuckson noted that, regardless of its cost effectiveness, prevention is of critical importance to making gains in public and population health.

While the participants highlighted a selection of particularly high-yield, cost-lowering strategies during the meeting, Mitchell and several others noted that many promising strategies, such as increased use of mid-level practitioners, additional ancillary providers (such as health coaches and nutritionists), salaried physicians, and a reassessment of the link between funding for medical education and hospital reimbursement, deserve further exploration and study as potential methods of lowering healthcare costs.

Attendees also explored the underlying notion of accountability as critical to improving the health of the nation and to creating a culture in health care that values efficiency and quality. They emphasized that all stakeholders in health must bear responsibility if the delivery system is to be reformed. For example, while Gilfillan and Toussaint suggested that providers bear responsibility for ensuring that care is delivered in the most efficient, safe, patient-centered manner possible, Mitchell added that patients are responsible for improving their engagement in the decision-making process. Without a mission and common understanding of collaborative engagement and accountability, Cutler noted that successful development and implementation of policies that address stakeholder concerns would fall short of their full potential.

Participant Leadership Responsibilities

Building on the idea of accountability, several attendees cited the need to identify specific entities that would assume primary responsibility for oversight of implementation and evaluation to ensure that the maximum potential savings were realized. Within the context of ongoing efforts to enact healthcare reform legislation, participants pointed to the public sector, including government at the local, state, and federal levels, as critical to providing oversight and ongoing support to the overall healthcare system infrastructure. Gilfillan stated that the role for government extended beyond the legislative branch to the executive branch as well. The Department of Health and Human Services and CMS were specifically viewed as setting important examples in payment reform and coverage, inasmuch as spending on the Medicare and Medicaid programs account for almost 40 percent of national health expenditures (CMS, 2009). Mitchell suggested that the increased provision of Medicare claims data as a public good to purchasers, plans, researchers, and the public would be a vital aid in analyses of cost and quality. Bailit termed the government, especially at the state and local levels, as critical to efforts at organizing providers and payers to affect changes in concert with ongoing national initiatives and in improving public and population health, including the physical and social determinants of health, such as education and community safety. In addition, several participants observed that state governments play a critical role in overcoming problems in commercial insurance markets through insurance regulation. For example, Rosenthal suggested that states could adopt all-payer regulations that could align the basic structure of pay for performance or risk-sharing methods in a marketplace.

Several participants highlighted the responsibilities that healthcare providers—ranging from nurses and physicians to acute, intermediate, and long-term care facilities—and commercial payers must bear to successfully reform the delivery system. For example, Tuckson cited the Healthcare Administrative Simplification Coalition, a collaboration between providers and payers to streamline administration by simplifying the credentialing process, standardizing data exchange, and leveraging health information technology. Providers, payers, and purchasers were also seen as playing important roles in improving patient health behaviors by encouraging preventive care and educating consumers on both the value of receiving care and the impact of individual health decisions on personal and population health.

Patients and consumers were also said to bear significant responsibilities for their care. Opportunities to participate in a shared decision-making process that stimulates patients to fully understand the risks and benefits of the diagnostic and therapeutic options specific to their clinical condition could increase consumer awareness of the value of alternative treatments, suggested Bailit, Mitchell, and Everett. In addition, consumers need to gain better understanding of the evidence indicating that more is not always better, suggested another participant.

Regardless of the specific stakeholder engaged, several attendees emphasized that none of these stakeholder groups should act in isolation without consideration of the other groups. It was suggested that affecting beneficial change requires the involvement of all sectors of the healthcare system, strong accountability, and agreement on the goals of improving quality and value.

NEXT STEPS FOR THE ROUNDTABLE

Although the ideas encapsulated throughout this summary reflect only the presentations, discussions, and suggestions that coursed throughout the workshops, and should not be construed as consensus or recommendations on specific numbers or actions, many of the thoughts and potential follow-up actions fall within the scope of the Roundtable mission and provide initial ideas for further Roundtable and field consideration, including the following:

- *Developing a strategic roadmap.* To apply the impressive and extensive information gathered throughout the various workshops, many discussed the need for a national strategic roadmap to identify the areas most likely to yield significant savings, the highest-priority strategies to realize those savings, and the specific steps needed to translate the potential into actionable recommendations that will result in truly lowered costs.
- *Improving the analytics.* While the estimates presented during the workshops represent initial steps in providing a sense of the relative amounts of inefficiency in the delivery system and the potential impact of key strategies, participants frequently emphasized that additional work will be required to refine and strengthen the accuracy of the numbers and their cross-cutting nature. Several additional facets suggested for consideration included specific delineation of estimates across the public and private sectors as well as the uninsured; consideration of areas of overlap between estimates, and of implementation and maintenance costs; and identification of the barriers to effective "spread" of successful strategies. In addition, the workshop presenters focused on the direct costs of health care, but the indirect costs of health care—ranging, for example, from those of absenteeism for unnecessary services to decreased investments in education—also warrant consideration.
- *Engaging multiple stakeholders.* Given the reality of abundant challenges and resistance to change, attendees observed that efforts to successfully control cost growth and lower spending while preserving innovation and outcomes could be achieved only with the cooperative efforts of the myriad stakeholders in health care— including patients, providers, manufacturers, payers, regulators, researchers, and policy makers, in both the private and the public sectors—aligned to improve insights, accelerate progress, and create a system grounded in delivering value to its constituents.
- *Informing health reform initiatives.* As efforts to reform the delivery system continue on both the federal and the local levels, specific attention was drawn to identifying inefficiencies in the healthcare system and the politically actionable policies to minimize them, because they carry paramount weight and clearly intersect with the goals of creating a value-based learning health system.
- *Enhancing transparency.* Building on the observations expressed by many about the lack of information as to the costs, outcomes, and value from health care, work to enhance the transparency of

system performance was viewed as particularly relevant for the Roundtable members, who represent the leadership of the key stakeholder sectors.

- *Focusing on strategies for more direct public engagement.* As heard throughout the workshops, the desire for information and engagement among health consumers has grown over the past few decades, yet the range of information exchange between the public and policy makers needs further development. Effective and efficient tools for translating technical language and information into accessible information for consumer use are required, as are methods of incorporating patient concerns and feedback into the policy decision-making process. Participants spoke of the role of education in clarifying the relationship between out-of-pocket costs and total medical spending, illustrating the impact of costs on all levels of society, and further motivating partnerships between consumers, providers, payers, and policy makers.

While the ideas summarized above reflect only the presentations, discussions, and suggestions that spanned throughout the workshops and should not be construed as consensus or recommendations on the specific numbers or opportunities, they provide informative insights into the opportunities to lower costs and improve outcomes present within the current healthcare delivery system, and represent areas needing further consideration. As these conversations continue, additional observations and suggestions are welcome and encouraged as the Roundtable continues to consider and explore these challenges and possibilities.

REFERENCES

Anderson, G. F., and B. K. Frogner. 2008. Health spending in OECD countries: Obtaining value per dollar. *Health Affairs (Millwood)* 27(6):1718-1727.

Anderson, G., and J. Horvath. 2002. *Making the case for ongoing care.* Princeton: Robert Wood Johnson's Partnership for Solutions.

Baicker, K., and A. Chandra. Medicare spending, the physician workforce, and beneficiaries' quality of care. 2004. *Health Affairs (Millwood)* Suppl Web Exclusives:W184-W197.

Berenson, R., J. Holahan, L. Blumberg, R. Bovbjerg, T. Waidmann, and A. Cook. 2009. How We Can Pay for Health Care Reform. The Urban Institute.

Brownlee, S. 2009. *Perception vs. Reality: Evidence-Based Medicine, California Voters, and the Implications for Health Care Reform.* http://www.effectivepatientcare.org/images/0909percent20CEPCpercent20Brownleepercent20Reportpercent20onpercent20EBM.pdf (accessed October 2, 2009).

Bureau of Labor Statistics. 2009. *Consumer Price Index-August 2009.* http://www.bls.gov/news.release/pdf/cpi.pdf (accessed October 2, 2009).

Casalino, L., S. Nicholson, D. Gans, T. Hammons, D. Morra, T. Karrison, and W. Levinson. 2009. What does it cost physician practices to interact with health insurance plans? *Health Affairs (Millwood)* 28(4):w533-w543.

CBO (Congressional Budget Office). 2004. *An Analysis of the Literature on Disease Management Programs. A Letter to the Honorable Don Nickles.* www.cbo.gov/doc.cfm?index =5909 (accessed 2009).

———. 2008. *Evidence on the Costs and Benefits of Health Information Technology.* http:// www.cbo.gov/ftpdocs/91xx/doc9168/05-20-HealthIT.pdf (accessed September 10, 2009).

Chandra, A. Personal communication: Costs of defensive medicine. December 20, 2009.

Chernew, M. E., R. A. Hirth, and D. M. Cutler. 2009. Increased spending on health care: Long-term implications for the nation. *Health Affairs (Millwood)* 28(5):1253-1255.

CMS (Centers for Medicare & Medicaid Services). 2009. *National Health Expenditure Data Overview.* http://www.cms.hhs.gov/nationalhealthexpenddata/01_overview.asp (accessed June 1, 2009).

The Commonwealth Fund. 2009. *The Path to a High Performance U.S. Health Care System: A 2020 Vision and the Policies to Pave the Way.* http://www.commonwealthfund. org/Content/Publications/Fund-Reports/2009/Feb/The-Path-to-a-High-Performance-US-Health-System.aspx (accessed August 26, 2009).

The Commonwealth Fund Commission on a High Performance Health System. 2007. *A High Performance Health System for the United States: An Ambitious Agenda for the Next President.* New York: The Commonwealth Fund.

Delaune, J., and W. Everett. 2008. Waste and inefficiency in the U.S. Health Care System clinical Care: A comprehensive analysis in support of system-wide improvements. *New England Health Care Institute.*

Devoe, J. E., A. Baez, H. Angier, L. Krois, C. Edlund, and P. A. Carney. 2007. Insurance + access not equal to health care: Typology of barriers to health care access for low-income families. *Annals of Family Medicine* 5(6):511-518.

DeVol, R., A. Bedroussain, A. Charuworn, K. Chatterjee, I. K. Kim, and S. Kim. 2007. *An unhealthy america: The economic burden of chronic disease charting a new course to save lives and increase productivity and economic growth.* Santa Monica: Milken Institute.

Docteur, E., and R. Berenson. 2009. *How does the quality of U.S. health care system compare internationally?* http://www.urban.org/UploadedPDF/411947_ushealthcare_quality.pdf (accessed October 2, 2009).

Elmendorf, D. W. 2009a. Letter to Honorable Nathan Deal.

———. 2009b. *Options for Controlling the Cost and Increasing the Efficiency of Health Care.* http://www.cbo.gov/ftpdocs/99xx/doc9911/02-25-Health_Insurance.pdf (accessed September 4, 2009).

Farnham, P. J. 2009. Insights from genomic profiling of transcription factors. *Nature Review of Genetics* 10(9):605-616.

Farrell, D., E. Jensen, B. Kocher, N. Lovegrove, F. Melhem, and L. Mendonca. 2008. *Accounting for the Cost of U.S. Healthcare.* McKinsey Global Institute.

Federal Bureau of Investigation (FBI). 2007. *Financial crimes report to the public: Fiscal year 2007.* http://www.fbi.gov/publications/financial/fcs_report2007/financial_crime_2007. htm#health (accessed September 11, 2009).

Fisher, E. S., D. E. Wennberg, T. A. Stukel, D. J. Gottlieb, F. L. Lucas, and E. L. Pinder. 2003. The implications of regional variations in Medicare spending. Part 1: The content, quality, and accessibility of care. *Annals of Internal Medicine* 138(4):273-287.

GAO (Government Accountability Office). 2008. Medicare Part B imaging services. http:// www.gao.gov/new.items/d08452.pdf (accessed March 1, 2010).

Greene, J., E. Peters, C. K. Mertz, and J. H. Hibbard. 2008. Comprehension and choice of a consumer-directed health plan: An experimental study. *American Journal of Managed Care* 14(6): 369-376.

Healthcare Administration Simplification Coalition. 2009. *Bringing better value: Recommendations to address the costs and causes of administrative complexity in the nation's health care system.* http://www.simplifyhealthcare.org/repository/Documents/HASC-Report-20090717.pdf (accessed October 1, 2009).

Hu, T., and G. Cohen. 2008. *Striking jump in consumers seeking health care information.* http://www.hschange.org/CONTENT/1006/1006.pdf (accessed October 2, 2009).

IBM Global Business Services. 2009. *CAQH CORE Phase 1 Measures of Success Study.* http://www.caqh.org/COREIBMstudy.php (accessed 2009).

IOM (Institute of Medicine). 2000. *To Err Is Human: Building a Safer Health Care System.* Washington, DC: National Academy Press.

———. 2001. *Crossing the Quality Chasm: A New Health System for the 21st Century.* Washington, DC: National Academy Press.

———. 2007. *Rewarding Provider Performance: Aligning Incentives in Medicare (Pathways to Quality Health Care Series).* Washington, DC: The National Academies Press.

Kaiser Family Foundation. 2009a. *Employer Health Benefits: 2009 Annual Survey.* http://ehbs.kff.org/pdf/2009/7936.pdf (accessed October 2, 2009).

———. 2009b. *Health Care Cost: A Primer.* http://www.kff.org/insurance/upload/7670_02.pdf (accessed September 7, 2009).

———. 2009c. *Kaiser Health Tracking Poll.* http://www.kff.org/kaiserpolls/posr022509pkg.cfm (accessed September 7, 2009).

Kindig, David, and G. Stoddart. 2003. What is population health? *American Journal of Public Health* 93:380-383.

Kutner, M., E. Greenberg, Y. Jin, and C. Paulsen. 2006. *The Health literacy of America's adults: Results from the 2003 national assessment of adult literacy.* http://nces.ed.gov/pubs2006/2006483.pdf (accessed October 2, 2009).

Lakdawalla, D. N., D. P. Goldman, and B. Shang. 2005. The health and cost consequences of obesity among the future elderly. *Health Affairs (Millwood)* 24 Suppl 2:W5R30-41.

Laveist, T., D. Gaskin, and P. Richard. 2009. *The economic burden of health inequalities in the United States.* http://www.laveist.com/uploads/Burden_Of_Health_Disparities_Final_Report.pdf (accessed October 1, 2009).

Menduno, M. 1999. Apothecary.Now. *Hospital Health Network* 73(7):34-38, 40, 32.

Milstein, A. 2009. *Tracking the contribution of U.S. Health Care to the global competitiveness of American employers and workers.* http://select.mercer.com/blurb/145847/article/20096311 (accessed August 7, 2009).

National Association of State Budget Officers. 2009. *Fiscal survey of states.* http://www.nasbo.org/Publications/PDFs/FSSpring2009.pdf/ (accessed September 7, 2009).

National Coalition on Health Care. 2008. *The Impact of Rising Health Care Costs on the Economy: Effect on Business Operations.* http://www.nchc.org/documents/Costs-Businesses-2009.pdf (accessed September 7, 2009).

National Guideline Clearinghouse. 2009. *National guideline clearinghouse.* http://www.guideline.gov/ (accessed October 2, 2009).

National Practitioner Data Bank. 2007. *2006 Annual report.* http://www.npdb-hipdb.hrsa.gov/pubs/stats/2006_NPDB_Annual_Report.pdf (accessed October 2, 2009).

Ngo-Metzger, Q., M. P. Massagli, B. R. Clarridge, M. Manocchia, R. B. Davis, L. I. Iezzoni, and R. S. Phillips. 2003. Linguistic and cultural barriers to care. *Journal of General Internal Medicine* 18(1):44-52.

Orszag, P. R. 2007. *Projected Financial Spending in the Long Run. Letter to the Honorable Judd Gregg, Committee on the Budget of the U.S. Senate.* http://www.cbo.gov/ftpdocs/82xx/doc8295/07-09-Financing_Spending.pdf (accessed September 4, 2009).

———. 2009. *Letter to the Honorable Nancy Pelosi.* http://www.whitehouse.gov/omb/assets/legislative_letters/Pelosi_071709.pdf (accessed October 2, 2009).

Partnership to Fight Chronic Disease. 2009. *About the issues.* http://www.fightchronicdisease. org/issues/about.cfm (accessed October 2, 2009).

Peterson, C., and R. Burton. 2008. *U.S. Health care spending: Comparison with other OECD countries.* http://digitalcommons.ilr.cornell.edu/keyworkplace/311 (accessed September 11, 2009).

Pollack, A. 2008. Patient's DNA may be signal to tailor medication. *New York Times,* December 29.

PriceWaterhouseCoopers. 2008. *The Price of Excess: Identifying Waste in Healthcare Spending.* http://www.pwc.com/us/en/healthcare/publications/the-price-of-excess.html (accessed September 20, 2009).

Rein, A. 2007. *Navigating health care: Why it's not so hard and what can be done to make it easier for the average consumer.* http://www.academyhealth.org/files/issues/Navigating HealthCare.pdf (accessed October 1, 2009).

Russell, L. B. 2009. Preventing chronic disease: An important investment, but don't count on cost savings. *Health Affairs (Millwood)* 28(1):42-45.

Smith, P. 2009. Enhancing clinical data as a knowledge utility. The Healthcare Imperative: Lowering Costs and Improving Outcomes Workshop, July 16-18, Washington, DC.

Thorpe, K. E. 2004. The medical malpractice 'crisis': Recent trends and the impact of state tort reforms. *Health Affairs (Millwood)* Suppl Web Exclusives:W4-20-30.

Tynan, A., A. Liebhaber, and P. B. Ginsburg. 2008. A health plan work in progress: Hospital-physician price and quality transparency. *Res Briefs* (7):1-8.

UnitedHealth Group. 2009. *Federal Health Care Cost Containment—How in Practice Can It Be Done?-Working Paper #1.* http://www.unitedhealthgroup.com/hrm/unh_working paper1.pdf (accessed October 19, 2010).

U.S. Department of Energy Biological and Environmental Research Program. 2009. *Exploring genes and genetic disorders.* http://www.ornl.gov/sci/techresources/Human_Genome/posters/chromosome/ (accessed October 1, 2009).

U.S. Census Bureau. 2009. *Income, poverty and health insurance coverage in the United States.* http://www.census.gov/Press-Release/www/releases/archives/income_wealth/014227.html (accessed October 1, 2009).

Valenstein, P., and R. B. Schifman. 1996. Duplicate laboratory orders: A college of American pathologists q-probes study of thyrotropin requests in 502 institutions. *Archives of Pathology & Laboratory Medicine* 120(10):917-921.

Wang, Y., and M. A. Beydoun. 2007. The obesity epidemic in the United States—gender, age, socioeconomic, racial/ethnic, and geographic characteristics: A systematic review and meta-regression analysis. *Epidemiologic Reviews* 29:6-28.

Wennberg, J. 2008. *Presentation: Evidence-based medicine: Vehicle to value efficiency?* http:// www.mtlf.org/docs/31177/Wennberg.pdf (accessed October 2, 2009).

Wennberg, J. E., E. S. Fisher, and J. S. Skinner. 2002. Geography and the debate over Medicare reform. *Health Affairs (Millwood)* Suppl Web Exclusives:W96-114.

The White House. 2009. *Fiscal Responsibility Summit.* http://www.whitehouse.gov/assets/ blog/Fiscal_Responsibility_Summit_Report.pdf/ (accessed September 4, 2009).

WHO (World Health Organization). 2009. http://www.who.int/social_determinants/en/ (accessed October, 2009).